TROWBRIDGE COLLEGE

BLYTH, Eric

Consultant Editor: Jo Campling

Social Work With Children: The Educational Perspective

Eric Blyth and Judith Milner

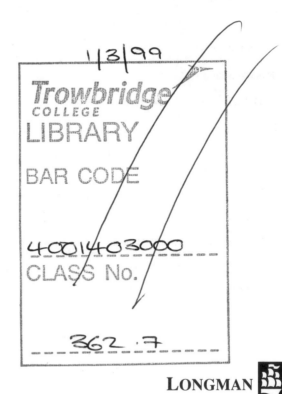
LONGMAN

London and New York

Addison Wesley Longman Limited
Edinburgh Gate
Harlow
Essex CM20 2JE
United Kingdom
and Associated Companies throughout the world

*Published in the United States of America
by Addison Wesley Longman, New York*

First published 1997

ISBN 0-582-29308-1

British Library Cataloguing-in-Publication Data

A catalogue record for this book is available from the British Library

Library of Congress Cataloging-in-Publication Data

Blyth, Eric
    Social work with children : the educational perspective / Eric Blyth and Judith Milner
        p.   cm.
    Includes bibliographical references (p.   ) and indexes.
    ISBN 0-582-29308-1
    1. Socially handicapped children--Education--Great Britain.
    2. Handicapped children--Education--Great Britain. 3. School social work--Great
    Britain. I Milner, Judith, senior lecturer.
    II. Title.
    LC4096.G7B59   1998   97-25031
    371.9'0941--dc21   CIP

Set by 7 in 10/11 Times
Produced through Longman Malaysia, CLP

CONTENTS

ACKNOWLEDGEMENTS

A number of friends and colleagues have helped us in a variety of ways in the writing of this book. First we wish to thank Jo Campling for her early encouragement, without whom this book would never have been more than just 'another good idea'. We also wish to thank our colleagues in the Centre for Education Welfare Studies at the University of Huddersfield for their continual support, for giving us ideas and the opportunity to discuss these, in particular: Sheila Baxter, Cedric Cullingford, Alan Dunkley, Dave Griffin, Alison Hodgson, David Hoyle, Tony Moore, Steve Stubbs, John Taylor and Joe Wilson.

In addition we wish to thank the long-suffering members of our families, Rosie, Beverley, Ian and Stuart, for their forbearance while this book was being written.

Eric Blyth and Judith Milner

ABBREVIATIONS

ACE	Advisory Centre for Education
ACESW	Association of Chief Education Social Workers
ADD	Attention Deficit Disorder
ADHD	Attention Deficit Hyperactivity Disorder
ADSS	Association of Directors of Social Services
AMA	Association of Metropolitan Authorities
AMMA	Assistant Masters and Mistresses Association
CACE	Central Advisory Council for Education
CCETSW	Central Council for Education and Training in Social Work
CNA	Carers National Association
DES	Department of Education and Science
DFE	Department for Education
DFEE	Department for Education and Employment
DHSS	Department of Health and Social Security
DSM	Devolved School Management
DOH	Department of Health
ESO	Education Supervision Order
ESW	Education Social Worker
EWO	Education Welfare Officer
EWS	Education Welfare Service
FAS	Funding Agency for Schools
GEST	Grants for Education Support and Training
GM	Grant-maintained
HMI	Her Majesty's Inspectorate of Schools
ILEA	Inner London Education Authority
INSET	In Service Education and Training
LEA	Local Education Authority
LMS	Local Management of Schools
NAS/UWT	National Association of Schoolmasters and Union of Women Teachers
NASWE	National Association of Social Workers in Education
NCDS	National Child Development Study
NSPCC	National Society for the Prevention of Cruelty to Children
NUT	National Union of Teachers
OECD	Organization for Economic Cooperation and Development
OPCS	Office of Population Studies and Census
OFSTED	Office for Standards in Education
PRU	Pupil Referral Unit

PSE   Personal and Social Education
RADAR   Royal Association for Disability and Rehabilitation
SCRE   Scottish Council for Research on Education
SHA   Secondary Heads Association
SOED   Scottish Office Education Department
SSI   Social Services Inspectorate
UPIAS   Union of the Physically Impaired Against Segregation

CHAPTER 1

The purposes of education and the growth of welfare

Introduction

The availability of free and compulsory education for its children is generally considered a hallmark of the development of a society and is emphasised as a basic right to which children should be entitled by the United Nations Universal Declaration of Human Rights and Convention on the Rights of the Child and the European Convention on Human Rights. However, while there is broad agreement that the purpose of education should be to prepare children for adult life, differing groups of people have placed differing emphases on the adult qualities desired. In the 1992 White Paper *Choice and Diversity* the government emphasises the moral dimensions of education's ability to shape future citizens: 'Regular attendance at school and taking advantage of a good education with a strong moral, spiritual and cultural context, are not only essential to becoming well qualified and growing up balanced, they are also one of the best deterrents against criminality' (DFE, 1992a, p. 6). The police, who could be expected to share this emphasis, demonstrate an equal interest in pupil safety. For example, a joint police/local education authority publication on curriculum liaison for responsible citizenship (West Yorkshire Police/West Yorkshire Local Education Authorities, 1988), views the police role in education with three- to nine-year olds entirely as one concerned with safety on the roads, in the home and near water, and with child abuse, leaving issues to do with inculcating respect for the law until the pupils are nine years old. Parents, who may well share the safety concerns of the police, are likely to emphasise education as preparation for successful participation in the world of work and protest strongly to schools about other pupils who disrupt their own children's academic progress. Pupils, on the other hand, are more likely to be concerned with the more immediate social realities of school, as the locus both of friendships and enmities and, in the case of extreme forms of the latter, expecting schools to protect them from bullying.

While there appears general agreement that education is a 'good thing', there has been no evidence of attempts to reconcile differences about the purpose of education. The history of the development of compulsory education in Britain reflects the differing emphases of various powerful groups which have influenced its avowed purposes: as a form of social control; promoting self advancement; and the means of providing a flexible labour force to meet the needs of the economy.

This chapter will examine the tensions arising from these conflicting aims not only in relation to the origins of compulsory education but also how they reflected subsequent debates. The complementary rise in welfare which accompanied a concern to deal with both 'deprived' and 'depraved' children will also be introduced and the scene set for the complex social issues which continue to test social workers in the educational context.

The origins of compulsory education in Britain

The development of formal compulsory education as a separate activity from education within the home under the influence of parents reflected power divisions in society. Although the power of the Church was to wane with the advent of industrialisation, until the late 1880s the major providers of formal education in Britain were the Church of England, the Roman Catholic and non-conformist churches and charitable bodies providing both day and Sunday schooling for children of the poor and of the very wealthy. These schools were characterised by strict discipline, emphasising the churches' focus on moral rescue and religious instruction. At the same time, the quality of teaching often left much to be desired: 'The master was often a man who had failed at other employment or was handicapped by some physical deformity' (Barnard, 1969, p. 3), indicating that teaching was not considered to be a highly skilled job which would demand universal respect.

These early themes of moral rescue and undervalued teaching permeate contemporary debates around education, the emphasis being on unruly pupils and inadequate teachers at times of civil unrest. Historically much has been expected of teachers in producing the 'right sort' of citizens with neither the skills required nor the purpose of the task being clearly articulated. It is here that the role of the teacher *in loco parentis* has its roots, with teachers – like parents – lacking support but receiving a large measure of criticism.

That state involvement in mass education did not occur earlier was the result of several factors including: the churches' unwillingness to relinquish their own powers as major providers of education; fears by non-established religious groups of interference from the established Church; the dominant political ideology of *laissez-faire*; resistance from employers at the prospect of losing a source of cheap labour; and similar resistance from parents at the prospect of losing the child's earnings (which for many would signify hardship of immense proportions); the shortage of teachers; and the costs to the state of providing education for all.

Although the strength of these sentiments did not themselves abate, there was a persistent pressure for increased state intervention in education. The common objective of compulsory state education was held by a variety of interest groups but with different motives and agenda. There was increased pressure from the poor themselves for access to education and the wherewithal to develop necessary skills to enable them to compete during a period of rapid industrialisation, coinciding with industry's need for a competent workforce. H. G. Wells wrote that: 'the Education Act of 1870 was not an act for common universal education, it was an act to educate the lower classes for employment on lower-class lines and with specially trained inferior teachers who had no university qualification' (cited in Coombes and Beer, 1984, p. 5).

A range of benevolent reformist pressures sought to 'improve' the working classes. The 'child-saving' movement had as its aim the liberation of children from oppressive working conditions and the preservation of their 'innocence' (Platt, 1969) but education of working-class children was not intended to be too extensive (Maclure, 1965) and there was also a view that children were in need of surveillance: 'Education was desirable because it prevented juvenile delinquency and mendicancy, because it increased a labourer's skill, productivity and earning power; because it prevented the growth of criminal classes; and because it led the workman to realize his true interests lay not in Communism or Chartism but in harmony with his employers' (Finer, cited in Carlen *et al.*, 1992, p. 19).

The value of compulsory education in ensuring that the working class learned to know their place – and stayed there – was a lesson quickly learned by the converts to 'enlightened self-interest' and one which has apparently not been forgotten: 'We are in a period of considerable social change. There may be social unrest, but we can cope with the Toxteths. But, if we have a highly educated and idle population we may possibly anticipate more serious social conflict. People must be educated once more to know their place' (DES official cited in Ranson, 1984, p. 241). The tension between education as a form of social control and a means of self-advancement and socio-economic mobility still remains. It clearly suits dominant socio-economic groups to hold out the carrot of self-improvement via education and the near-mythical figure of the self-made (wo)man as evidence that the system does reward those who are worthy and who make sufficient effort and that, conversely, failure to succeed is the result of individual rather than institutionalised shortcomings.

The development of compulsory education

The introduction of compulsory education in Britain was itself a gradual process. Although the Elementary Education Act of 1870 is conventionally regarded as the hallmark statute, its immediate effect was to do little more than plug the gaps in provision left by voluntary educational bodies and church schooling. It provided for the administration of education by local School Boards who were given powers to provide and maintain elementary schools from public funds. Full-time school attendance was not universally compulsory but Boards were given powers – if they wished – to introduce by-laws to compel attendance and to impose financial penalties on parents who failed to make proper arrangements for their children's education. In practice there was a national shortage of school places and considerable regional variations in local by-laws, the enforcement of parents' statutory obligations and arrangements for exemptions from attendance. Early graduation from school was legitimated by the acquisition of specified standards of educational proficiency. For example, the London School Board passed a by-law making attendance compulsory for children aged between five and thirteen years, but a child who had achieved a prescribed level of educational attainment was allowed to leave school at the age of ten years, while younger children adjudged to be 'beneficially and necessarily' at work were permitted to attend half-time only. Neither did the 1870 Act ensure *free* elementary education for all, although Boards were authorised to waive the school fees of children from impoverished families. School attendance officers did not always implement this legislation rigorously (for an overview, see Rubenstein, 1969) and magistrates also took a lenient view of truancy. Nevertheless, the introduction of the 1870 Act not only began the inexorable push for free compulsory schooling it also signalled a significant shift in the way in which children were perceived, their new relationship with education replacing that which they had previously had with employment. Prior to education legislation, earlier mines and factories legislation required minimal provision of education and school attendance as a condition of the employment of children. The Factory Act 1844, for example, permitted children over eight years of age to be employed half-time in workshops and factories and at thirteen they could be employed full-time. The 1874 Factory Act raised these ages to ten and fourteen years respectively. Two years later the 1876 Education Act prohibited the employment during school hours of children living more than two miles from an elementary school who were aged under ten years and of those between ten years and fourteen years unless they had reached certain specified educational targets. Children in rural areas were also permitted to be absent from school for up to six weeks so that they could assist with agricultural work. Rural traditions of children assisting with harvesting were responsible for the summer vacation during July and August. The aspirations of those who had sought to rescue children from oppressive working conditions were subjugated to the needs of the economy. While child employment during school hours was increasingly proscribed, the interests of employers and poor families meant that many children were forced to work before and after attending school. The employment of school-age children has continued to raise educational concerns and has contemporary relevance as a child protection issue, a topic to which we return in chapter 10.

The Education Act 1880 increased the upper age limit of compulsory education to ten years, although there was still no statutory regulation of how attendance was to be controlled or enforced, nor by whom. In 1899 the upper age of compulsory education was further increased to twelve years and by the end of the century most elementary school fees had been abolished (although the complete elimination of fees for elementary schooling had to wait until 1918). The Education Act 1902 increased the age of compulsory education to a child's thirteenth birthday and abolished *ad hoc* school boards, placing the responsibility for education provision on education authorities under the auspices of county and county–borough councils and enabling the running costs of voluntary (church) schools to be met from taxation and local rates revenues. However, although there was an obligation on local authorities to provide education, there remained widespread variation throughout the country because provision of education other than elementary was a discretionary power and not a statutory duty for councils of non-county boroughs with a population exceeding 10,000, and for urban districts with a population exceeding 20,000 at the 1901 census.

The 1918 Education Act finally abolished half-time schooling and raised the school leaving age to fourteen, at which it remained until 1947, when it was raised to fifteen, and was further raised to sixteen in 1972. However, because of continuing unresolved tensions between education as a means of self-advancement yet responding flexibly to the needs of the economy, the effective policing of compulsory education has always been perceived as problematic: 'The difficult thing would not be to pass a law making education compulsory; the difficult thing would be to work such a law after we had got it' (Matthew Arnold cited in Maclure, 1965, p. 82).

Enforcing school attendance

By the beginning of the 1900s, official records indicate 88 per cent of children under twelve years were on school rolls, although average daily attendance was only about 72 per cent. While attendance figures are now generally higher, little appears to have changed in the intervening period concerning the main reasons for absence, these still consisting of poverty, availability of juvenile employment, weather conditions, domestic duties and alternative attractions (Digby and Searby, 1981). However, then – as now – knowledge of attendance rates assumes accurate recording of registration. Throughout the nineteenth century grants to schools and reimbursement of teachers were dependent on pupil numbers and levels of attendance as well as pupil attainment in formal examinations. While the report of the Newcastle Commissioners in 1861 did not fully endorse the concept of 'payment by results' it did acknowledge the need for effective accountability in schools and in the 1880s more than a third of a head teacher's salary and more than a fifth of the salary of an assistant teacher were related to pupil numbers and attendance (Rubenstein, 1969). Payment by results did not disappear until the turn of the century. Much as contemporary concerns surround the accuracy of school attendance registers to minimise the prevalence of 'unauthorised' absence (see chapter 7), there was thus a strong incentive for schools to under-report absence.

As we have indicated above, early enforcement of attendance was both patchy and variable. Apart from the variable strength of opposition from families and employers, Carlen *et al.* (1992) observe that selective targeting was based on judgements about whether greater advantage would accrue from certain children continuing in domestic or industrial labour, especially if this relieved the state of providing financial support to families. Because of their higher visibility boys were more likely to be the focus of official intervention than girls whose absence tended to be associated with low-profile activities such as household, child-care and other domestic duties (Green, 1980).

The School Boards were empowered to appoint officers to enforce attendance. Stevenson and Hague (1954) outline the duties of an 1870s School Attendance Officer as:

- ensuring that the name of every child between the ages of five and fourteen years (unless previously exempted from attendance at school according to law) was on the register of a public elementary school, or to satisfy themselves that the child was under efficient instruction in some other manner;
- securing the regular and punctual attendance at school of children whose names were on the school roll;
- making enquiries and reporting with regard to the remission of school fees in necessitous cases and applications for part-time labour certificates.

Those appointed as school attendance officers tended to be middle-aged men who had previously been employed in the police or armed forces, a trend which continued well into the twentieth century and which has been at least partly responsible for the continuing authoritarian image of the education welfare service (Blyth and Milner, 1988). However, it would be a mistake to regard such recruitment practices as unique. The Victorian precursor of the Probation Service actively recruited former police officers, while other early recruits included a complete bench of magistrates and the chief constable of Liverpool. Despite being appointed because of an 'authoritarian' background, officials in all these settings shared a common missionary ideal, seeing themselves as the saviours of the 'deprived' as well as the 'depraved'. Although the central focus was on attendance enforcement, school attendance officers were well aware of the impact of poverty and material disadvantage on access to educational opportunity. Robert Aitken, an early president of the attendance officers' national association stated: 'Those with whom we are in contact require our sympathy and all our counsel. Children brought up too often in poverty and squalor and huddled in wretched homes, what thought have they for good education. School life can never succeed, or the influence of school, while home life is cramped and crushed by insanitary and often immoral surroundings' (cited in Coombes and Beer, 1984, p. 6).

The mottoes selected for the two national associations in education welfare at the end of the nineteenth and the beginning of the twentieth centuries respectively ('Children: these we serve' and 'For every child a chance') indicate the welfare, rather than the purely attendance enforcement, orientations of officers' work. Education welfare is the oldest welfare service established by the state and the roots of modern social work, with its emphasis on child-centred interventions, are to be found in accounts of its inception. Despite subsequent policy reforms and the impact of financial constraints many of these functions remain and half a century after Aitken's pronouncement a Superintendent Attendance Officer was able to assert: 'Few vocations offer more scope for real social service' (Education, 1946).

The state, education and the family

The introduction of compulsory education marked a significant change in the relationship between children and work but it also had important ramifications for the relationship between children and their parents. Carlen *et al.* (1992) note that this is central to the debate about how education should best respond to the needs of industry and commerce.

The introduction of compulsory education and imposition of sanctions against parents who failed to secure their children's 'proper education' represented a significant dilution of the rights of parents over their children, not in favour of children themselves but in favour of the state. While education legislation did, and still does, allow for a child's exemption from registration at a school on the grounds that (s)he is being educated 'otherwise', very few parents are in a position to make alternative education provision other than in school. For most children, compulsory education effectively means compulsory schooling. When a child is in school, therefore, both responsibility and control are transferred from parents to the school. The legal definition of a teacher's duty while *in loco parentis* was established in the 1890s and outlined by Lord Esher (then Master of the Rolls) as a duty 'to take such care of his boys as a careful father would take care of his boys' (Williams *v* Eady, 1893). Subsequent legal decisions have determined that the concept of 'reasonable care' should be applied in the context of school rather than that of the home. A further point to be made – as illustrated by court action over corporal punishment in British schools prior to its abolition in state schools – is that so long as courts have been satisfied that a teacher has behaved 'reasonably' while acting *in loco parentis*, parents cannot over-rule their actions, however much they disapprove.

By handing over at least partial responsibility for their children to the state, schooling has also become a means by which families may be subject to scrutiny and surveillance by the state. Not only has school become a prime vehicle for the identification of poor children, undernourished children, potential victims of child abuse, young carers etc. but family life itself is much more amenable to examination. Indeed, the fact of compulsory attendance has itself become a proxy measure of parental competence. Not only was the introduction of compulsory education accompanied by the provision to apply financial penalties to parents who failed to ensure their children were properly educated, child care legislation has meant that measures of compulsory care can also be imposed via the courts. Under the provisions of section 1(2)(e) of the Children and Young Persons Act 1969 (which formed the substantive basis of child care legislation in England and Wales before the Children Act 1989) one of the grounds on which a child could be deemed as being in need of 'care or control' was that (s)he was 'of compulsory school age ... and is not receiving full-time education suitable to his (*sic*) age, ability and aptitude and to any special educational needs he (*sic*) may have'. If a court wished to impose a care – or any other – order it also had to be satisfied that the child was 'in need of care and control which he (*sic*) is unlikely to receive unless the court makes the order'. Beginning in the early 1970s this legislation was exploited by the juvenile court in Leeds who used adjournments – and the ultimate threat of removal from home if school attendance didn't improve – to compel children to go to school (Berg *et al.*, 1977, 1978). By the early 1980s nearly four times as many children were in local authority care under Section 1(2)(e) in Leeds compared to the country as a whole (Bowen, 1985). What became known as the 'Leeds scheme' was adopted by many juvenile courts despite considerable criticism (e.g. House of Commons, 1984; Blyth and Milner, 1987a). One of the more telling indictments of the scheme was made by a Principal Education Welfare Officer undertaking a research study which specifically focused on a group of young people who had been committed to local authority care following failure to attend school. Despite the fact that educational problems had been directly responsible for their admission to care, Bowen (1985) concludes that not only had this produced no educational benefit at all but that the lives of these young people had been significantly disrupted and damaged by the experience. Despite a stout defence of the scheme's integrity and legality by its architects (e.g. Hullin, 1985, 1988; Berg, 1996), their 'artificial use' of care pro-ceedings was partially instrumental in creating the pressure for legislative reform which saw the replacement of the Children and Young Persons Act with the Children Act 1989.

The scope for local authority and court intervention in family life where children were not attending school was given greater force following a High Court judgement (*Re* DJMS, 1977) in which Lord Denning ruled that the fact that a child was not attending school was sufficient to satisfy the 'care and control test' for care proceedings. This ruling had wider repercussions than simply facilitating state intrusion into the families of children who were not going to school. Because the care and control test in respect of Section 1(2)(e) proceedings was considered easier to prove than any of the other grounds for care, it was widely believed that many children found their way into local authority care through this route when the real concerns about their welfare more appropriately focused on grounds whose existence would be more difficult to prove to a court, such as 'neglect' or 'moral danger'.

Although we discuss the legislative framework concerning school attendance in more detail in chapter 7, it is pertinent to note here that a 1992 court ruling (*Re* O, 1992) effectively re-applies the ruling of *Re* DJMS in relation to the imposition of a care order under the provisions of the Children Act 1989. In considering an appeal against the making of a care order, the court ruled that extensive non-attendance at school itself demonstrated that a child had suffered 'such an impairment of educational, social and intellectual development' that warranted the imposition of a care order and that 'where a child is suffering harm in not going to school and is living at home it will follow that either the child is beyond her parent's control or that they are not giving the child the care that it would be reasonable for the child to receive'.

The introduction of the Parents' Charter (DES, 1991a; DFE, 1994a), though explicitly encouraging parents to become 'active partners' with their children's schools and teachers, also serves as a reminder of their responsibilities and the very real limits on their power to influence both educational resourcing and what goes on in school.

Schools and access to welfare

Various statutes have afforded recognition to the welfare aspects of education, including an eventual redesignation of attendance officers as education welfare officers in the 1940s – a title which remains in most parts of England and Wales, although the designation 'education social worker' has since been adopted by a number of local authorities. The establishment of universal compulsory education meant that schools soon came to be seen as suitable locations for the delivery of other welfare services, including the provision of clothing, milk and lunches and some health services. For example, the Education (Provision of Meals) Act 1906 was introduced because of concerns that some children were prevented by malnourishment from taking full advantage of education.

Later, state interest in children's welfare grew as a result of concern about the health of children during and between two world wars. Rose (1985) charts the rise in the measurement of children in schools – their weights and heights, IQ and health status. It became possible to collect comparable information on a large number of subjects and subsequent analysis led to the construction of norms. Developmental norms represented not only what was 'normal' for children at any given age but also enabled the 'normality' of any individual child to be assessed by comparison with norms. Although much of this measurement of children had its roots in a desire to improve the health status of deprived children, reflecting the shared ideologies of both health professionals and the early welfare workers, the development of norms enabled applied and clinical psychology to psychologise what were social factors. The translation of social problems into individual, psychological problems had the effect of shifting the emphasis of social work away from interventions aimed at rescuing children from poverty and into individual casework (for an overview, see Darbu, 1991).

As the twentieth century progressed the role of schools in the welfare network became increasingly evident. A series of government reports (CACE, 1963, 1967; DHSS, 1968) recognised the strategic location of schools in detecting at an early stage children experiencing disturbance and distress and playing an active part in the treatment and monitoring of 'social casualties'. Theoretically since all children aged over five would be attending school their absence could itself indicate that welfare or other assistance might be required. The Plowden Committee (CACE, 1967) recognised the potential contribution of social work in combating underachievement in schools and recommended the establishment of a school social work service to complement the work of teachers. Although the full role of school staff in dealing with child abuse took some time to become established (Milner and Blyth, 1988; see also chapter 10), the opportunity provided teachers for detecting potential abuse was recognised, the Seebohm Committee noting: 'We cannot emphasise our view that the role of teachers is of prime importance. It is he or she who, seeing the child daily in class is often the first to become aware that all is not well' (DHSS, 1968, p. 64). Nearly two decades on, though, this was a message that still had not been absorbed: 'It is with the child that has not so far come to the notice of Social Services that the school has a vital role to play. Too many children, we suspect, have not been observed as potential victims of child abuse, either at all or because no one is spotting the symptoms' (London Borough of Brent, 1985, p. 155).

As evidence of the differential effect of schools on various aspects of their pupils' lives (including behaviour patterns and exposure to delinquency) became more apparent, so did the debate about the relative impact of a range of influences on children's behaviour intensify. These issues are discussed more fully in the next chapter before we look more closely at the development of welfare in the context of the education reforms of the 1980s and 1990s.

CHAPTER 2

The impact of school

Introduction

Measuring the impact of school on pupils' subsequent performance as adults in society depends upon at least minimal levels of agreement as to what effects education should have on pupils. As we have shown in the previous chapter, the aims and purposes of education are as diverse as the pressure groups able to influence education provision to their own ends and, despite their relative powerlessness, the responses of the immediate consumers of education themselves. The complex interplay of the numerous agenda in education will be examined in this chapter with reference particularly to the way in which pupils' social agenda influence academic agenda but also take into consideration other aspects of power which impact on pupils such as class, gender and 'race'.

Whatever emphasis is placed on the purpose of education, school impacts on pupils in a number of ways which have long-term effects and it offers the main alternative environment to the family during a period of significant physical, intellectual, emotional and social development. School offers pupils the opportunity to learn far more than they are formally taught, consisting of much more than teachers teaching. It is a complex social organisation which will exert far-reaching influences on children whether they are in or out of it. The physical environment of this society impacts strongly on children in a way which is so obvious that it is often ignored. School is a physical alternative to the home but one which provides little of interest for pupils to explore (Claxton, 1984), nor is necessarily clean and tidy or busy and interesting (Clegg and Megson, 1976). A school and its playground are curiously private yet lacking in privacy for both pupils and teachers. That it shuts itself off from the outside world will be testified by parents bewildered on parents' evenings by the problem of identifying which is the front door before struggling to find their way about the building. Accessibility at other times is no more straightforward especially for schools taking seriously the need to protect pupils and staff from unwanted and potentially dangerous visitors.

Although most pupils become accustomed to the physical environment of school, they soon learn that teachers cannot provide protection in many parts of the building, particularly the lavatories, the playground and that strange territory – the journey between home and school – where neither parents nor teachers hold influence over events.

In these places, children are in charge and there are opportunities for child–child interactions which have the potential for either fun or misery. This is the unofficial world of school to which Measor and Woods (1984) refer as the informal peer group culture of school which might or might not fit with the formal culture of the school as encompassed in the goals and aspirations of the school, linking to what is officially taught. While much of the literature focuses on the negative effects of anti-school and delinquent peer groups (for an overview, see Cullingford and Morrison, 1997), there is also a substantial body of information on the benefits to pupils of belonging to a peer group.

Because there are links between the development of social understanding, logical reasoning and moral judgement (Bee, 1985), the formation of friendships influences the formal culture of school. For example, emotional and intellectual development is linked to positive peer group membership (Dunn and Maguire, 1992; Rosenthal, 1993) thus enabling pupils to participate in the academic curriculum more effectively. Social competence is also affected as many of the skills, attitudes and beliefs acquired in early playground interactions transfer to other situations (Slukin, 1981) with children learning to initiate, discuss, influence and change rules, learn rituals, avoid conflict and make contracts. As self-efficacy levels become stable by junior school age, the successful negotiation of the playground is as important as the successful negotiation of the classroom. Children's self-image and self-evaluation are more strongly influenced by the informal culture of school (Fine, 1980), particularly in the case of black children (McAdoo and McAdoo, 1985; Mac an Ghaill, 1988). Similarly, gender identity is predominantly established in the playground, with boys defining themselves early by preferring sex-segregated and larger groups for play (Galton *et al.*, 1980) in which they learn to resolve disputes by reference to 'the rules' whereas girls develop a style of interacting in smaller groups where they are prepared to abandon disputed games to maintain friendships (Gilligan, 1982). Thus, the playground is hardly a breeding ground for the construction of 'new men'.

Friendship groups act as important sources of support and security at times of need (Measor and Woods, 1984), providing protection from bullying in particular. Later friendship groups in adolescence are not necessarily anti-school and anti-family. Indeed, it has been argued that they provide a sort of surrogate family (Brown, 1987), particularly where positive family relationships are absent (Sletta *et al.*, 1996). The purpose of school to induct pupils into adult life is achieved to a large extent by the informal culture of pupils' social relationships with children learning under what rules of behaviour others operate in similar circumstances, what are merely parental quirks in control and discipline, and what are universal, social and moral norms (Foot *et al.*, 1980).

Thus, both unpopular and absent pupils – whether through truancy or exclusion – may not only be placed in increased physical and emotional danger (Cohen and Hughes, 1994; Lewis, 1995) but they are lacking support from friends of a positive nature. Slukin (1981) described children who do not 'fit in' socially as children who are in a rut, unable to experiment in new games, new situations or find ways out of difficulties. They do not learn the rules for joining groups and experiences of hostility from other children discourage them, disadvantaging them in their social relationships from an early age.

Levels of bullying in schools are difficult to assess accurately (e.g. Olweus, 1979) although it appears to be more common in primary schools with up to a quarter of pupils reporting experiences of which about one in ten is persistent. Although the rate drops in secondary school to about one in twenty-five, bullying incidents in secondary school appear to be more serious (Smith and Sharpe, 1994). Without the support of a positive peer group, persistently bullied children become 'legitimate' victims (Arora and Thompson, 1987). Children who persistently bully are also a group with difficulties. As with their victims, they have poorer school attainment but they are more likely to grow up to become physically violent and delinquent (Smith and Sharpe, 1994). While Stephenson and Smith (1987) found bullies to be generally unpopular, there is some evidence that male bullies gain some popularity with girls as a result of their activities (Olweus, 1979).

In summary, pupils who fail to negotiate the informal culture of school are unlikely to be any more successful in the formal school culture, but teachers are handicapped in their endeavours to compensate for this by the simple fact that they cannot penetrate the informal culture easily and have limited knowledge of it (Chapman *et al.*, 1979; Slukin, 1981). However, the behaviour of children in the classroom is highly dependent upon the behaviour and perceptions of teachers. What a teacher expects of a pupil is not necessarily what the child is capable, or deserving, of, as teachers make assessments of pupil potential on the basis of class, gender and 'race' factors as well as intellectual criteria. We discuss these in more detail later in this chapter but the point we wish to make here is that teacher perceptions tend to be both self-fulfilling and long-lasting in their effects. While Rosenthal's and Jacobsen's (1968) early research into self-fulfilling prophecies has been largely discredited, other studies do point to the subjectivity of teachers' assessments of their pupils (for an overview, see Pilling and Kelmer Pringle, 1978).

Effective schools

The effects of schools on their pupils as both children and adults have been extensively studied, the consistent finding from the research being that pupils' academic progress varies greatly according to the school they attend. The first major study (Rutter *et al.*, 1979) revealed that differences between school outcomes were not simply due to the nature of their intakes or the social and family backgrounds of their pupils but to factors operating within the school. Academic achievement was linked with pupil behaviour in terms of school attendance, discipline and delinquency. Smith and Tomlinson (1989) studied 25 multiracial comprehensives, finding that there were dramatic differences between the schools despite catchment areas and that the 'school effect' was greater than Rutter and his colleagues suggested. Additional support for the school effect comes from a study of progress in inner London primary schools which found that schools were four times as important as family background in accounting for progress in the early school years (Mortimore *et al.*, 1988a). Although attainment is heavily influenced by home background, progress was more likely to be influenced by schooling, with primary school effects being greater and longer lasting than secondary school effects (Goldstein and Sammons, 1995).

School effects, whether for good or ill, persist into adulthood, although not necessarily in a direct way. For example, Gray *et al.* (1980) followed up the schools in the original Rutter study, finding indirect continuities to be strong. Pupils at the less effective schools were twice as likely to be poor attenders at school and were twice as likely to leave school without educational qualifications. The school leavers without qualifications were twice as likely to go into unskilled work and twice as likely to have poor employment records (for a detailed discussion of the connections between childhood experience and adult life, see Rutter and Rutter, 1993). These are discussed more fully in chapter 7 but we make the point here that pupils with behavioural problems are more likely to become the adult clients of social workers. On the other hand, effective schools exerted a beneficial effect on all pupils. Those who had a positive school experience differed from others in that they were more likely to exert planning in relation to both work and marriage – not feeling at the mercy of fate, thus helping the development of positive self-esteem and self-efficacy.

Various research studies, conducted in a number of different countries, have shown that positive school experiences can not only provide support to children in adverse social circumstances but even help to counter their impact. For example, pupils' feelings of 'belonging' to the school offered a measure of protection against adolescent substance abuse (Hawkins, Catalano and Miller, 1992). Similarly, Botvin (1995) has identified the value of schools' life skills training programmes in reducing pupils' subsequent drug use. Fergusson and Lynskey (1996) observed a correlation among school-age children between their professed enjoyment of school and their resilience to adverse social circumstances. In a study of female survivors of sexual abuse Romans *et al.* (1995) note the positive value of these young women's enjoyment of school. The authors comment that success in the social, academic or sporting life of school appears to offer some measure of protection from the long-term effects of abuse and traumatic family relationships, the latter observation endorsing Werner's (1990) view of school providing a refuge from a 'disordered household' and Wallerstein's and Kelly's (1980) research illustrating the role of school in supporting children whose parents' marriage was ending. These findings appear to reinforce Rutter's cautious assessment of the protective effect of schooling as probably 'critically important only in subgroups under stress and with a lack of other positive experiences' (Rutter, 1991a, p. 8).

Overall, effective schools are up to 32 per cent better than average (for an overview, see Rutter and Rutter, 1993), therefore it is vitally important to understand what makes for an effective school in terms of both positive social experience and good cognitive performance. The Rutter *et al.* (1979) study echoed much of what Clegg and Megson (1976) had commented upon earlier about the characteristics of good schools: that schools need to be clean, tidy, busy, interesting, stimulating and democratic places; the ethos being of much more importance than factors such as type of intake or school size.

Unfortunately it is not easy to translate the research findings into workable policy. Three schools which attempted to implement the findings of the Rutter research (1979) managed only modest accomplishments (Rutter *et al.*, 1986). The main reasons for this were lack of external pressure for change, lack of change in key staff positions and inadequacy of long-term strategies. Further studies were undertaken of secondary schools which not only served socially disadvantaged populations but were also in considerable trouble, had poor community reputations and had appointed a new head at the time of crisis. Two of the schools experienced considerable improvement over a five-year period despite the intake remaining the same. These improvements reflected moves towards purposeful leadership, involvement of staff and pupils, clear expectations for everyone at the schools and an atmosphere that was constructive and enjoyable. Rutter and Rutter (1993) comment that the climate must be ripe and considerable skills are needed to bring about change in effectiveness of schools.

Gray (1994) identifies three main factors in school effectiveness. First, schools need a visible ideology so that pupils as well as staff can give a reasonably clear account of what school is about. Second, that teachers expect pupils to achieve and pupils find themselves being stretched and, third, that there is not only an absence of conflict between teachers and pupils but some sort of positive rapport. These factors do not just happen, they are 'managed', so school leadership becomes more important than was previously understood. The identification of these factors as important and the relative unimportance of resourcing does not mean that resource issues can be ignored (see, also, Sammons *et al.*, 1995 for an excellent overview).

Ensuring adequate resources for a school and their effective deployment would be part of the effectiveness of leadership. This may be particularly important for schools at the lower margins of success. For example, at the Ridings School, Halifax, lack of resources and failure to employ existing resources effectively emerged as one, although not the only one, of the major contributing factors to the school's spiral of decline (BBC, 1996), although the use of existing resources, as opposed to insufficient resources, received more prominence in the inspectors' report ordered by the Secretary of State

(OFSTED, 1996a). Reynolds makes the important point that: '. . . some effectiveness factors that come out of the study of effective institutions may be the *result* of effectiveness rather than the cause and the ineffective school simply may not be able to generate them', suggesting that it may be necessary to be directive with ineffective schools on the grounds that: '. . . people who have collectively permitted a school to hit educational rocks are unlikely be able to steer it off them' (Reynolds, 1996, p. 51).

Although the desired qualities of effective school leadership have not been as well researched as overall school effectiveness, it is possible that at least one of the skills involved will be an understanding of the complex interactions between teachers, pupils, parents and ancillary staff. Teacher expectations of pupils may be high but can only too easily be thwarted if no attention is paid to the role of the school caretaker. The effectiveness of whole school strategies which utilise the skills of the wide range of adults in a school and support services have been well demonstrated (Gill and Monsen, 1996).

A whole school approach has three principal characteristics. First, pupil behaviour and attendance are not simply regarded as functions of individual personality or external forces such as peer, family or neighbourhood pressures. The potentially significant influence of the school community – including governors, all staff, pupils and parents – and school processes are also recognised. Second, accountability for valuing good behaviour and attendance is owned by the school's senior management and shared by all members of the school community and not seen as the exclusive responsibility of specialist pastoral and welfare staff. This commitment manifests itself in designated behaviour and attendance policies and – in many schools – the introduction of computerised systems for the collection and analysis of attendance data. Third, all features of school life, including curriculum and school 'ethos' – and not only specific behaviour and attendance policies and procedures – are recognised as contributing to the promotion of good behaviour and attendance.

The Education Reform Act 1988 has made the role of parents in supporting school endeavours more clear. However, gaining all parent and community support is far from easy, being unfortunately most problematic in the instances of 'difficult' pupils whose parents who do not readily visit school. Kavanagh (1989) complained that teachers make assumptions that 'difficult' pupils have 'difficult' parents but this is a two-way process. There exists substantial research to show that the parents of the most disadvantaged pupils – local authorities in their role as parents of 'looked after' young people – are often disinterested in schooling (see chapter 5 for a fuller discussion).

There has also been an emphasis on wearing school uniform to create belongingness rather than as a means of sterile discipline. However, it is not easy to create a genuine ethos of belongingness in schools which have a traditional bias towards meeting the needs of middle-class, white boys. The effects of this on pupils from lower socio-economic classes, minority ethnic groups, and girls is discussed below in terms of their educational opportunities and their need to engage in sophisticated survival strategies.

Social class

The general thrust of research shows that the higher a person's social class of origin, the greater their chance of achieving high educational qualifications and vice versa (see, for example, Rutter *et al.*, 1979), although the absolute achievement in basic skills of working-class pupils in the most effective schools studied by Mortimore *et al.* (1988a, b) was higher than those of middle-class pupils in the least effective schools after three years of education. However, quite how class affects achievement is not so well understood, with researchers emphasising different aspects of the school process (see, for example, Gillborn and Gipps, 1996). Teacher attitudes and expectations are also cited as factors with teachers underestimating working-class children's language competence (Wells, 1984) and assessment of their reading ability (Southgate, 1981). Tizard *et al.* (1988) found that the abilities of pupils from lower socio-economic groups were underestimated regardless of 'race' or gender. While Dusek and Joseph (1983) maintain that teacher expectations are a major factor, a small number of researchers e.g. Croll (1981), have found no social class effect.

Mortimore *et al.* (1994) point to a more complex process operating in teachers' underestimation of pupils from a working-class background. For example, they suggest that teachers may be picking up on cues about pupils such as eligibility for free school meals or physical appearance – and found that pupils from homes where the father was absent were perceived as having a greater incidence of behaviour problems. As behaviour and attainment are linked, the causal effect becomes even more complicated. It does appear that some teachers have different expectations of pupils from different backgrounds, irrespective of cognitive performance, but this effect on attainment may not be as great as that of poverty.

With changes in employment patterns which challenge traditional conceptions of clearly distinct working- and middle-class groups, it might be more difficult to replicate earlier studies but there has been an insidious growth of child and family poverty. Since 1979 there has been a considerable rise in the proportion of the population living in poverty, although the rise in overall poverty has been accompanied by a disproportionate rise in the numbers of children and families affected by poverty. The proportion of children living in families with less than half the average national income, after housing costs, rose from 16 to 33 per cent between 1981 and 1992. Inequality of income is greater in the UK than in other northern European countries (OECD, 1995). The growth and impact of child and family poverty has been hidden to some extent by rhetoric about deliberate 'welfare motherhood' and a political climate which encourages the view that such families could do better if only they tried harder. However, the reality of some families' poverty is highlighted when the very real gains made by some groups are examined. A 24 per cent increase in the real annual income of the average household since the late 1970s conceals a 40 per cent increase enjoyed by the richest 20 per cent while the income of the poorest 20 per cent fell by 5 per cent (Townsend, 1991; Mintel, 1994). Actuarial evidence indicates that the wealth gap is set to widen further (Johnston, 1994). Such differences would not necessarily be significant if evidence of the much-vaunted 'trickle down' effect was less elusive. However, there is evidence that poverty contributes to high levels of stress within families which may well affect children's behaviour and performance in schools (Rutter, 1991a, b; NUT, 1992; AMA, 1995; OFSTED, 1995a). The experience of life on the poverty line in 1990s Britain was graphically illustrated by a children's charity, NCH: Action for Children (1994), which claimed that a family reliant on Income Support could not afford the diet fed to children living in a Bethnal Green workhouse in 1876.

Although teachers may hold differing expectations of pupils depending upon social class factors, this is by no means the largest source of unequal treatment in schools. The single biggest determinant of teacher behaviour is the pupil's gender.

Gender

Historically, girls in primary schools have settled more easily into the classroom, achieved better academic results and scored lower on rates of maladjustment (Davie et al., 1972). It was suggested that the female role was perhaps easier for girls in primary schools than the male one for boys, with a notion developing that the primary school was a feminised environment which favoured girls at the expense of boys. However, there exists an assumption that girls' early superiority will fade with time, allowing boys to 'catch up' naturally (Whyte, 1983), and a closer look at classroom organisation and activity reveals that boys are given precedence in almost every area of school life (Esposito, 1979; Cook and Campbell, 1981; Mortimore et al., 1994).

Girls' achievements are often disparaged by teachers as products of hard work rather than talent (Acker, 1981) and girls develop perceptions of their success based on these early responses. For example, girls underestimate their potential as writers (DES, 1985) although they consistently outperform boys on assessment of writing (DES, 1986a). Murphy (1994) suggests that, for girls, almost all the negative commentary they receive is directed at the intellectual quality of their work and that this affects their academic self-image. Boys, on the other hand, are more likely to be criticised for lack of effort and given remedial work (Whyte, 1983). Thus, they do not become as discouraged as girls by their failures and tend to over-estimate their chances of success (Licht and Dweck, 1983).

The day-to-day organisation of school favours boys, whether this is by registering their names first (Kelly, 1981), the use of books with a masculine bias (Buswell, 1981; Winter, 1983), or the regular requests to girls to undertake domestic duties such as pencil sharpening (Tizard *et al.*, 1988). While it is important to cherish instances of differences between girls and boys and respect their wishes to be treated differently, teacher attitudes and school organisation is such that sexual harassment becomes an ordinary event in primary schools (Mahoney, 1985), with the gender loading of secondary school language rendering girls subordinate in the day-to-day interactions of both classroom and playground (Lees, 1986). Tizard *et al.* (1988) found that white girls, in particular, were invisible to their teachers while Foster (1988) highlights the double dilemma for black girls whose harassment is both sexist and racist. White girls are controlled by the term 'slag' but black girls have to endure both 'slag' and 'wog'.

Primary school acts, therefore, as a way in which boys are prepared for the overtly masculine environment of the secondary school at which it is expected that their 'natural' superiority will be displayed and where they will cope easily with the sarcasm and bantering of the teacher-dominated classroom. Here, boys will be challenged by teachers to encourage greater critical analysis but responses to girls will be more neutral or their questions will be taken as indicating a lack of understanding rather than intellectual curiosity (for an overview, see Delamont, 1994a, b).

Educational research has shown, surprisingly, that girls have increasingly survived the masculine environment of secondary schools, steadily improving their academic performance, particularly where they are educated separately from boys (Smith, 1989). The most obvious conclusion to reach from the research in gender inequality in education is to teach girls separately and ensure that they have effective teachers who are committed to equal opportunities. But this leaves us with the problem of boys who seem to need to dominate girls to achieve their maximum potential. It would be hard to charge teachers with being the sole custodians of equal opportunities, school being but one part of the process by which boys become men: 'We need a conception of male and female subcultures as related, two parts of a single unitary phenomenon. Just as masculine and feminine are complementary parts of a single gender system, so girls' and boys' subcultures are in reality only two aspects of one subculture, with different implications for the sexes' (Cockburn, 1987, p. 43).

For boys, the psychological construction of masculinity is rooted in the social context of men's power relations to women (Hearn, 1996) and the dominance of boys in the classroom and teachers' academic expectations of them is but one part of becoming masculine. The informal culture of the school is also important with boys dominating in the playground via the development of macho identities and controlling girls via sexual descriptions of their (supposed) behaviour (see, for example, Lees, 1986; Mac an Ghaill, 1994). And it is not unreasonable to suppose that for boys who find it difficult to achieve domination through academic success, the informal culture of the school will become a more important environment for the making of their masculine identities. Teachers attempting to deal with disruptive boys need to understand that boys' agenda will be wider than a simple resistance to teacher authority, their behaviour being tied up with girls' behaviour out of the classroom.

Girls, particularly in adolescence, are relatively under-researched in comparison with boys. Delamont (1994b) argues that this is because researchers are tempted by the bizarre and exciting not the respectable and conventional and adolescent boys' resistance is seen as more threatening to teachers. McManus (1995) argues that girls are more respectable and conventional, dismissing 'troublesome' girls in schools in only two pages. Davies (1984) found that girls were unconformist mainly in respect of rules to do with not smoking and wearing school uniform, misdemeanours which come low on teachers' lists of offences compared with 'constant irritation to class and teacher' (Blyth and Milner, 1996a). Mac an Ghaill (1994) found girls' resistances to be more covert than boys', with much faked compliance so that when girls' more overt resistance brought them to the attention of teachers, this was seen as an act of individual deviancy.

He also found that the psychological construction of femininity was more complex than that of boys and we suggest that this is because the social context of power relations in which they must operate requires a sophisticated understanding of the intricate negotiations needed for survival – meek submission being not a preferred strategy. Girls have long-term views of their feminine identity which transcend the simple choice in school between getting a 'good education' or getting a boyfriend. Their view of adulthood includes getting a job which gives them opportunities their mothers lacked; one which acts as a potential marriage market; and one in which they can get away from 'men bossing them about' (Mac an Ghaill, 1994). To survive in the social reality of modern womanhood, they need to negotiate the formal and informal cultures of school as they affect girls as potential wives, mothers and workers.

Girls' behaviour in the informal culture of school is also of relevance to teachers' understanding of boys' resistance. While girls go to great lengths to avoid the term 'slag', they do display an attraction for 'Macho Lads' which Mac an Ghaill (1994) found had unintended outcomes for teachers' relations with anti-school boys. Their relations with these boys were more sophisticated than their teachers realised – they did not value hypermasculinity in itself but perceived it as a legitimate defence against authoritarian male teachers. This has particular implications for understanding African Caribbean masculinity in schools which is influenced by both gender and 'race' effects.

'Race' and ethnicity

It is a common assumption that black children inevitably fare badly in a white education system. The Rampton Report (1981), for example, suggested that the negative performance of minority ethnic pupils might be affected by low teacher expectations due to negative stereotypes about such groups of pupils' abilities. This view receives further support from evidence about the disproportionate number of African Caribbean pupils excluded from school (Blyth and Milner, 1996b), placed in schools for pupils with learning difficulties (see, for example, Tomlinson, 1981, 1982; Wright, 1990), and in special units for children with emotional and behavioural difficulties (Cooper *et al.*, 1991). Not all the research evidence points to a straightforward causal link between prejudice and low attainment, however, and we should be wary of over-generalising the relationship between ethnicity and educational experiences and performance. In particular the significant differences in achievement among different ethnic groups should be recognised (e.g. the Swann Report, 1985). An ILEA (1990) study of educational attainment of Year 11 pupils based on 1987 examination results concluded that children of Bangladeshi, African Caribbean and Turkish origin obtained results significantly below those of other groups. However, after taking account of gender, verbal reasoning scores on entry and characteristics of the schools attended, children of African Caribbean, English, Scottish and Welsh origin were performing least well. In keeping with other studies, the results also pointed to the differential impact of different schools on the educational attainment of children from different ethnic backgrounds.

Regarding racism in schools as a single entity overlooks the resilience of some minority ethnic groups of pupils and extrapolates inaccurately from primary school studies. Gillborn and Gipps (1996) say that the situation is too varied for simple talk of 'black under-achievement'. For example, the changing ethnic population of schools in the 1990s showed that although pupils of Black African background often achieve relatively higher than their peers of African Caribbean origin, this is complicated by differences in social class and gender. Similarly, Indian pupils consistently achieve more highly than pupils from other South Asian backgrounds and, in some areas, white pupils but again class – and its association with language competence – may well be a factor. However, it is clear that African Caribbean young men in particular appear to be achieving considerably below their potential, and black pupils, on average, have not shared in the increasing rates of educational achievement (Gillborn and Gipps, 1996).

Language is a major factor in African Caribbean educational disadvantage. Gibson and Barrow (1986) noted that while Asian pupils routinely receive extra assistance with language problems neither African Caribbean pupils nor their teachers expected such remedial help, mistakenly assuming the existence of a common language. Gillborn (1990), however, notes that while the use of patois by African

Caribbeans is an important symbol of ethnic identity, within the school system it may be seen by teachers as threatening and confrontational.

Despite early disadvantage, at sixteen years African Caribbean pupils' academic results were better than those for white pupils (Kelly, 1988) with these pupils reversing the trend for white pupils with black girls outperforming black boys. This reversal of the trend for white pupils in the 1980s has been explained in terms of characteristics of black mothers, Rutter (Spencer, 1982) citing better assistance with homework in black households as a factor, Driver (1980) citing recognition of the realities of black motherhood, the Bristol Child Health and Education study (1986) associating reading attainment with mothers' social class and age. Additionally, Channer (1995) has found a correlation between strong religious affiliation and educational achievement. These studies seem to rest on stereotypes of strong black mothering and it is dangerous to assume that black mothers can always compensate for institutionalised oppression and structural inequalities (see, for example, the report into the death of Tyra Henry (London Borough of Lambeth, 1985)).

Mirza (1992) argues that it is erroneous to make assumptions about black motherhood on the basis of the disproportionate number of black lone-parent families. Her study showed that 78 per cent of black families have two parents and that a significant number of lone-parent families were headed by a lone father – a factor not found in white lone-parent families. Phoenix (1991) regards black lone-parent families as a positive and strategic lifestyle and the trends in white girls' success at O and A level perhaps indicate that they too are beginning to follow a black pattern of being anti-school in subtle ways but not anti-education, as discussed in the earlier section on gender effects.

The danger in overestimating the positive qualities of black motherhood is that African Caribbean boys become increasingly pathologised with teachers influenced by stereotypes existing in the wider community which views black masculinity as somehow problematic and threatening. Brandt (1986) found that teachers were more likely to perceive African Caribbean pupils as truculent and Asian pupils as conformist while Mac an Ghaill (1988) revealed teachers extending the stereotype of conformist, middle-class Asian pupils to all Asian pupils.

Westwood (1990) demonstrates how African Caribbean masculinity is exoticised, with boys falling into either the 'sporting hero' or 'feckless and irresponsible' category – the latter seen as somehow dislocated from family life. The sporting hero stereotype is further influenced by the fact that African Caribbean children are more likely to make use of sports facilities than whites and Asians (DES, 1986a), with low-achieving African Caribbean boys participating more in extra-curricular sporting activities at school. Success in sport as a career is elusive and teachers who encourage their black pupils to direct their efforts into sport may well limit their academic aspirations (Carrington, 1986). Additionally, the presence of low-achieving black boys on the sports field holds the potential for increasing group rivalry in differing school 'territories'.

This can increase racial tensions in schools and contribute to racist harassment. Macdonald *et al.* (1989) stress the importance of understanding the impact of peer culture in the development of racism, arguing that male violence cannot be separated from the culture of racism. As we have suggested in the previous section, boys may well develop hypermasculinities in the informal culture of school to compensate for under-achievement in the classroom. Where these underachievers are also African Caribbean pupils and therefore more susceptible to criticism from teachers about their behaviour (Tizard *et al.*, 1988) they are likely to be perceived by teachers as potentially 'dangerous' (for an excellent overview see Gillborn and Gipps, 1996).

Conclusion

The impact of school on its pupils is life-long, affecting not only their subsequent employment careers but also their adult social performance. However we determine the ideological purposes of education, effective schools should enable their pupils to fulfil their academic potential and survive the school's informal culture regardless of race, gender or social class. It is especially important for schools to compensate children from unhappy, unsatisfactory homes as the school effect is crucial in these instances. While isolating pupils with problems from mainstream schooling can be justified as offering immediate benefits for both school and pupils, this ignores the role of school processes in creating and ameliorating the problems which pupils may experience, thus ultimately reducing the overall effectiveness of schools. Individualising pupil problems also affects the development of welfare systems supporting schools, limiting the role of social workers and reducing the development of whole school approaches. We discuss the implications of this more fully in chapters 3 and 4.

CHAPTER 3

Education reform in Britain

Introduction

In common with other developments in social policy, the period since 1979 in Britain has been characterised by an explicit attempt on the part of government to introduce market forces to public service provision. A notable aspect of this has been the privatisation of public utilities such as energy supplies and transport. In other areas of public service, such as education, the surge of the market has stopped short of management buy-outs and the wholesale disposal of publicly owned assets. Nevertheless the education reforms of the 1980s and 1990s have exerted a marked impact on the provision of education and the relationship of the education system to various interest groups within the community. These reforms have had the effect of not only increasing the marginalisation of disadvantaged pupils but seriously threatening the entire welfare network.

Although the major education reforms of the late twentieth century have been sponsored by successive Conservative administrations, officially expressed concerns about the failure of the post-war state education monopoly to provide equality of access to education and its inefficiency pre-date the succession of Conservative Party administrations between 1979 and 1997. It is generally agreed that the so-called 'Great Education Debate' was launched following a speech delivered by the then Labour Prime Minister James Callaghan at Ruskin College, Oxford, in 1976, in which he expressed concerns about the impact of progressive tendencies in education, the failure of education to meet the needs of industry and the need for a common national curriculum.

At that time there was evidence of broad political consensus on the need to improve the quality of education in terms of its responsiveness to industrial and commercial demands and consensus on education as a means to combat disadvantage had not yet disappeared. Whitty and Menter (1989) note that when the Conservatives won the general election in 1979 there was little to indicate the radical policies that were to come over the next few years. In political terms the early Conservative education policies were more in keeping with the 'Old Tories' than with 'New Right' liberal marketeers and privatisers. For example, the introduction of the Assisted Places Scheme, although allowing for the transfer of academically able pupils from the state to the private sector at public expense, was more a response to the reduction of a style of education increasingly unavailable in the state system through comprehensivisation than the encouragement of private education *per se*.

The education market in Britain

The 'creeping privatisation' approach to education policy characteristic of the early post-1979 Conservative administrations was abandoned in favour of more radical market-oriented policies, initially under the provisions of the Education Reform Act 1988 and subsequently the Education Act 1993 in England and Wales and parallel, although not identical, legislation in Northern Ireland and Scotland. Such differences account, at least in part, for the different impact reform has had on Local Education Authorities in England and Wales, Education and Library Boards in Northern Ireland and Regional and Area Councils in Scotland. The contraction of the role of English and Welsh LEAs while increasing both central government powers and school autonomy has been more pronounced than for their Northern Irish and Scottish counterparts. (For an overview of education reform in Northern Ireland and Scotland see, for example, McKeown *et al.*, 1996 and Arnott *et al.*, 1996 respectively.)

Although the essential tenet of the education market is that excellence can be best achieved by increasing parental choice through bringing competition and the style of the market place into education, other agenda (not least one of cutting costs) have militated against total de-regulation and the untrammelled operation of the free market.

According to its proponents the key elements of the British education market are: choice, information, autonomy, accountability and quality control and diversity.

Education reforms have ostensibly increased parental influence over their children's education through membership of school governing bodies; increased choice of which school to send their children; and given them the opportunity to decide whether the school attended by their children should 'opt out' of local government control by becoming grant-maintained. In Northern Ireland the drive to increase parental influence was more muted for several reasons. Much secondary education was already selective on the basis of academic ability. Compared to the rest of Britain there was also a proportionately larger voluntary school sector consisting of voluntary grammar schools and Catholic-maintained schools (McKeown *et al.*, 1996). In Scotland different factors were in operation, Brown (1996) highlighting greater rural isolation; a general commitment of parents and professionals to education at the local comprehensive school and, with the exception of Edinburgh, a much smaller independent education sector, as pressures exerting resistance to an English- and Welsh-style education market. What should also not be overlooked is that while the Conservative Party formed the majority political party in Westminster, its representation at both national and local government levels in Northern Ireland and Scotland has been much lower, therefore compromising its mandate to enforce unpopular changes.

In England and Wales the Education Act 1980 provided for parental representation on the governing body of each LEA maintained school and the Education (No. 2) Act 1986 increased the number of parents on schools' governing bodies. The Education Reform Act 1988 increased significantly the powers of governing bodies which had previously been largely restricted to general oversight of the curriculum and school organisation. The 1988 Act gave governors increased powers over budgets and financial control, appointment of staff, discipline, oversight of the National Curriculum, pupil assessment, religious education, collective worship, admission and exclusion appeals, collection of school performance data, and whether the school should seek grant-maintained status. However, Deem (1996) argues that it would be erroneous to see in the increased involvement of parents of schools' governing bodies and governing bodies' increased powers and responsibilities a substantial step in the direction of 'parent power'. School governors are primarily white, middle-class and highly educated (Keys and Fernandes, 1990), while co-opted, and especially LEA, governors, rather than parent governors, play the major role in running schools because of their external contacts and positions in local networks.

Education reform and parental choice

Under the provisions of the Education Act 1980 and supported by subsequent legislation, parents have the right to 'express a preference as to where they would like their children to go to school'. If this preference is not met the LEA must provide an explanation. It is important to note, given the rhetoric about parent choice, that their legal right is to 'express' a choice. They do not have an unequivocal legal right to exercise that choice.

Among market advocates there is an assumption that: 'In the market-place all are free and equal, differentiated only by their capacity to calculate their self-interest' (Ranson, 1990, p. 15). Differences are legitimated by pathologising those who make 'poor' choices or who do not make choices at all as 'bad' parents, with little recognition of the impact on the ability to pursue self-interest of what Bourdieu and Passeron (1990) describe as 'cultural capital'. Parents with 'cultural capital', who have knowledge of schools, are able to interpret schools' promotional material and performance data, are able to 'work the system' (using such strategies as making multiple applications, applying for scholarships, using appeals procedures, even moving house to be nearer a preferred school), are able to present a positive image of themselves when negotiating with key gatekeepers and are able to provide transport for children to travel to a school of choice, will be in a better position to maximise their choices.

Despite the rhetoric of parental choice there is increasing evidence that, in the deregulated market, schools are choosing their pupils, the Audit Commission (1996a) reporting that 20 per cent of children did not attend their parents' 'first choice' school, and parents expressing low levels of satisfaction with the choices they are able to make. There is also increasing evidence of schools excluding 'undesirable' (i.e. high-cost/high-risk/low-achieving) pupils and reluctance to accept pupils excluded from other schools – an increase at least in part fuelled by pressure on schools to demonstrate positive (popular) images. Usually such practices take place out of the glare of publicity, although proof of their existence – if not necessarily an accurate indication of their prevalence – is revealed by the instances which occasionally receive a high profile in the media (e.g. Manton Junior School in Nottinghamshire and The Ridings School in Halifax, where teachers threatened to take strike action to enforce the exclusion of disruptive pupils).

Events at Manton Junior School revealed another aspect of the exercise of parental power (in default of real parental power) and which is also usually hidden from public view, where some parents may force the removal of an unpopular child by threatening to remove their own children from the school.

Effective parental choice depends on substantial spare capacity in the school system. While the 1988 Education Act introduced the concept of 'open' enrolment, preventing both schools and LEAs limiting admissions below the school's full capacity, at the time of publication of the 1992 White Paper *Choice and Diversity* the government claimed that there were about one and a half million surplus places in British schools. An explicit role of the education market is to reduce this spare capacity, parental choice identifying the unpopular schools which will be targeted for closure (although in reality, parents – including those whose children attend ostensibly 'failing' schools, as well as small, uneconomic rural schools – have invariably resisted closure). Nevertheless a clear expected outcome of market forces, therefore, will serve to reduce the scope for the exercise of parental choice.

Legislative measures under which a school may acquire grant-maintained status provide for limited parental rights. Only parents whose children are on roll at the time of any ballot have the opportunity to determine whether the school becomes grant-maintained and, once a decision to opt out has been taken, there are no provisions for a subsequent ballot to opt back in to LEA control. For future parents of children at a school which has already become grant-maintained the decision will already have been taken.

School autonomy and accountability

It is axiomatic that the exercise of informed choices depends on access to accurate information. All schools within the state system are required to publish annual details about the curriculum provided, the performance of pupils in public examinations, the progress of pupils at the end of each Key Stage of the National Curriculum, rates of absence, exclusions and school leavers' destinations. Such information is presented in the form of local and national 'league tables' designed to enable parents to make better informed decisions. In practice the publication of 'league table' performances has not been without its problems. There has been considerable debate about the appropriateness both of the choice of performance indicators themselves and the methods of their measurement, the latter illustrated by the controversy over the use of 'raw' or 'adjusted' data. Government ministers were keen that 'raw' data should be used, since they were suspicious that 'adjusted' data would provide schools with an opportunity to 'fiddle the statistics'. Such suspicions were supported by Professor Harvey Goldstein of London University who is quoted as saying: 'If schools are going to publish their exam results, I would put a health warning over them saying "read this at your peril"' (cited in ACE, 1995, p. 16). However, the use of 'raw' data is not neutral in its impact as it favours those schools able to be more selective about their intake.

Although the government's view prevailed, the first such table for examination results, published in November 1992, was immediately criticised for its lack of accuracy and validity, while the DFE itself expressed concern over the recording and interpretation of 'unauthorised absence' when performance data for school absenteeism were published in 1993 (see also chapter 7). On BBC News, John Patten (then Secretary of State for Education) responded to criticisms that many schools had refused to send in their absence data: 'What I am worried about is that these schools which have refused to send the information have got something to hide,' and warning that he would be 'sending in the inspectorate to find out what is going on' (Patten, 1993).

Although Patten's replacement as Secretary of State for Education (and subsequently embracing the Employment portfolio also) appeared to adopt a more conciliatory approach towards educationalists, recognising that: 'there is, of course, a great deal that comparative tables *cannot* tell us. Many of the qualities that make up a good school or college are difficult to quantify or distil into a percentage. . . . Performance data can never be conclusive in itself' (Shephard, 1994), the publication of such data remained controversial. In the summer of 1996 the National Association of Head Teachers advised its members (most of whom were head teachers in primary schools) to ask their governing bodies not to submit the results of tests taken by eleven-year-old pupils, which would form the basis of the first set of performance tables for primary schools, and complaints about their accuracy and validity surfaced even before the results were publicised in early 1997.

Significantly, league table performances inevitably underplay general improvements in standards and emphasise the relative placing of schools within them. They also fail to take account of the progress an individual pupil may have made during their school career and, unless account is taken of the nature of the school's intake, the real measure of progress at pupil or school level may not be reflected in formal examination results and league table positions. Whatever general progress has been made, there will always be 'top-of-the-league' and 'bottom-of-the-league' positions and these are the ones which will figure in public (and parental) perceptions of school performance. And any improvements made by a school placed at or near the bottom of the league table risks being lost in the context of general improvements in the criteria for published performance. The extent to which energies might be diverted mechanistically towards league rankings is evidenced by Clare (1993) quoting the head teacher of an independent boys' secondary school: '(parents) were very keen to see the school move up the league table because it makes them feel their money is being well spent'.

The narrowness of the criteria on which school performance is measured is largely a factor of what is readily quantifiable. Notably those features of school life which are less easily measurable, such as teaching quality and the nature and the quality of pupils' learning experiences, do not feature in the published performance data. Neither do the arrangements for collecting and analysing data distinguish between those features which are within the school's control and those which are not. Furthermore they do not provide any indication of 'added value' – the contribution the school makes to pupil progress and achievement (McPherson, 1992).

The education reforms of 1988 and 1993 promised increased autonomy for schools. For schools remaining within the local authority sector this would be achieved through the devolution to schools of an increasing proportion of the total education budget and increased powers and responsibilities for governing bodies ('Local Management of Schools' in England and Wales and 'Devolved School Management' in Scotland). Under these arrangements funding for individual schools is based on the number of children on roll and is age-weighted to take account of the different costs of educating different-aged children. The funding formula also allows for additional costs regarding provision for children with 'special educational needs'. The resources available to a school are, therefore, a direct reflection of pupil numbers and, it is assumed, of the school's popularity with parents.

More radically, education reforms provided parents with the opportunity to determine whether the school attended by their children should opt out of local political control altogether and acquire grant-maintained status, thereby receiving funding direct from the government, assuming increased freedom and responsibility and being able to seek from the Secretary of State a change in the school's character. The then government promoted the idea of increased autonomy as a principal attraction for schools of its reforms: 'The Government firmly believes that self-government is best for state schools' (DFE, 1992a, p. 19); 'Schools that have opted out have welcomed the new sense of ownership and independence. They can decide what they want to do and get things done without having to ask permission from the Town or County Hall. They are able to spend more in the classroom. Many schools become more popular with parents after opting out' (DFE, 1992b, p. 2). Indeed, former Secretary of State for Education John Patten described grant-maintained status as the 'natural organisational model for secondary education' (Patten, 1992). However, despite financial inducements from the government, the rate of opt-out has been variable both geographically and between the primary and secondary sectors, much slower than anticipated and is showing signs of slowing down. Only 1,158 out of a total of 24,000 schools in England and Wales (approximately 5 per cent of the total) had opted out between September 1988 when opt-out was introduced and March 1997 (Hamilton and O'Reilly, 1997). Opting out has proved more popular among secondary schools compared with primary schools with 16 per cent of secondary schools opting out while only 2 per cent of all primary schools have done so (DFE, 1995a). Parents' evident reluctance to grasp the 'opportunity' of independence more enthusiastically led the then Prime Minister John Major to announce his government's proposal to scrap parental opt-out ballots for all voluntary-aided (i.e. church) schools, of which only 350 out of 4,032 had opted out up to October 1995 (Charter, 1995). According to the proposal such schools would automatically opt out unless their governing bodies insisted on remaining with the LEA. While the combined opposition of both Anglican and Roman Catholic bishops forced the government to abandon these plans, the very fact that the government contemplated such measures at all is indicative of the limited commitment to parental choice. A further indication of the previous government's limited commitment to parental choice regarding the status of schools is revealed by the comments of Kenneth Clarke, erstwhile Secretary of State for Education: 'If I'd been Secretary of State in 1988, I would not have put in this balloting system. . . . They [ballots] remain the biggest single obstacle in the way of moving to grant-maintained status' (cited in Hamilton and O'Reilly, 1997). Despite the rhetoric, early research into grant-maintained schools in England indicated that there was little evidence of increased parental involvement in grant-maintained schools although grant-maintained status could enhance the power of the head teacher (Power *et al.*, 1994, 1996). (See also chapter 8 for a discussion concerning grant-maintained schools and exclusions.)

The price of increased autonomy for schools is increased accountability (which for grant-maintained schools and their governing bodies includes legal liabilities previously the responsibility of the LEA) and procedures for quality control. Mechanisms for ensuring account-ability and quality control include: publication of performance data in school prospectuses; annual report to parents by governing bodies; independent inspection of schools via OFSTED; and teacher appraisal/ assessment.

In addition to these planned mechanisms of accountability there appears to be increasing recourse to the courts to expose schools' failings and secure compensation for unsatisfactory standards. In one instance a London borough made an out-of-court settlement of £30,000 to a twenty year old who claimed he had been bullied at school years previously. In another case a twenty-five-year-old man is claiming compensation from the London Borough of Bromley after being excluded from school at the age of six and subsequently receiving no education for three years (Carvel and Dyer, 1996). Two teenagers who had been pupils at schools which had been formally designated as 'failing' schools following inspection by OFSTED have also initiated legal action claiming their examination results had been adversely affected because of the school's poor standards (O'Reilly, 1996a).

No diversity, no choice

Conservative governments expressed enthusiasm for the development of different types of school, and schools have been encouraged to develop special areas of interest, e.g. partnerships between schools and business. However, the drive towards diversity has been considerably mitigated by the centralised imposition of uniformity, notably through the prescription of the National Curriculum to be followed by all pupils in state schools (although private and 'public' schools are exempt from the requirement to follow the National Curriculum).

Determining the nature of the National Curriculum is clearly a political exercise, as recognised by former education minister Michael Fallon. He claimed that without 'political interference' from ministers: 'We would have seen history redefined as current affairs, geography covering politics not places, and English shorn of grammar but including Monty Python' (Fallon, 1992).

At school level there has been little evidence of either diversity or innovation. Indeed, despite the new discourse of specialisation, where grant-maintained schools have sought to change their character, this has most frequently been to 'introduce' academic selectivity (hardly surprising since this is the most efficient way of scoring highly in the performance tables): 'The vast majority of GM schools exhibit a reinvigorated traditionalism which is as likely to lead to uniformity as to foster innovative diversity' (Power *et al.*, 1996, p. 108).

Centralisation

Although much has been made of the impact of education reforms on 'liberating' schools by reducing the powers of and removing altogether those agencies which are identified as inhibiting or distorting market relationships, these reforms have replaced local democracy with massive centralisation and increase in powers of the Secretary of State. Critics on both the political left and right have not failed to highlight this. Green (1993) – an ardent free-marketeer – opposes the National Curriculum as a measure which both alienated teachers and placed the government at their mercy. Rather he maintains the government should have made parents true partners in education, not merely outsiders judging schools, and schools would have been more prepared to cooperate with parents. For Green 'the tendency of the Thatcher and Major governments . . . has not been to widen the scope for human creativity, but to increase central control' (Green, 1993, p. 141).

The increased powers of central government are largely exercised through quangos to which appointments are made by the Secretary of State and to whom appointees are accountable. The operation of quangos is rarely accessible to public scrutiny and accountability. Although quangos have played an important role in British public life for many years, under successive Conservative administrations they have assumed increased powers in recent years and by 1994 controlled nearly 20 per cent of all public expenditure. At the same time the political composition of quangos has changed dramatically through the government's reduction of the role of locally elected members and their replacement, by and large, by individuals known to be supportive of the Conservative Party (Cohen, 1994; Cohen and Weir, 1994; Weir and Hall, 1994).

Within education major quangos have been created to perform tasks previously performed by LEAs. For example, the Funding Agency for Schools (FAS), established in 1994, is not only responsible for administering funds to all grant-maintained schools but also shares responsibility with the LEA for school administration where the proportion of GM schools in a particular LEA area is between 10 and 75 per cent. The FAS will replace LEA functions entirely if more than 75 per cent of schools in a particular local authority area become grant-maintained. Members of the FAS come from a variety of backgrounds and a significant number are not educationalists. The FAS has a specific brief to promote opting out and will also have responsibility for school closure, irrespective of parental wishes and previous local democratic processes; pupil numbers; ensuring that there are sufficient school places; and ensuring that every child of compulsory school age is being educated. By March 1997 the FAS had shared responsibility in 8 LEA areas for the primary sector and in 49 LEA areas for the secondary sector. In 3 LEA areas (all outer London boroughs) the FAS had complete responsibility (personal communication).

The 1988 Education Act gives the Secretary of State additional powers to remove the governing body of a 'failing' school and replace it with an Education Association which will have the powers and funding of a governing body of a GM school. The Education Association will manage the school(s), with powers to sack staff and responsibility to: 'revitalise the leadership and management of the school', until such time as the Secretary of State is satisfied they have achieved a satisfactory level of performance. At the end of the period under the Education Association, the school(s) will be considered for GM status. If the Education Association fails in this task the school will close, the eventual fate of Hackney Downs School in London (O'Connor *et al.*, 1997).

The 1993 Education Act severely curtails the role of Local Education Authorities. The government envisaged that, as the number of GM schools increased and a bigger proportion of the education budget transferred to local authority schools, LEAs would become 'mainly providers of services to schools' (DFE, 1992b). LEAs will retain specific, largely welfare, responsibilities for providing an education welfare service; an educational psychology service; organising home-to-school transport (although this will be opened to competition); any remaining maintained schools; the costs of premature retirement and dismissal; assessment and statementing of children with 'special educational needs'; enforcement of school attendance and liaison with Social Services Departments; provision of non-school based education for 'children who behave badly' (and replacing previous powers with duties to make such provision). In relation to other services provided by the LEA the government will not allow it to retain staff and operate any services 'which go beyond what it requires for the efficient exercise of its own functions within its own area. LEAs may only trade at the margin of capacity' (DFE, 1992a, p. 32). Increasingly, the government expects such services to be provided by the private sector. Local authorities are no longer required to establish an education committee. Eventually 'some local authorities may soon be in sight of no longer needing them' (DFE, 1992a, p. 32).

Critique of the education market

Free-marketeers have criticised the state monopoly in education for creating 'winners' and 'losers'. However: 'Markets derive their efficiency from the fact that there are winners and losers, risk-takers and bankruptcies, entrepreneurs and uncertainty' (Veljanovski, 1990, p. 6), and Keith Joseph (Conservative Secretary of State for Education between 1981 and 1986) claimed that 'one of the main virtues of privatisation is to introduce the idea of bankruptcy, the potential of bankruptcy' (cited in Ball, 1990, p. 63).

However, if market advocates consider as unacceptable the existence of 'winners' and 'losers' under a state monopoly is their survival in the market system any more acceptable? What is significant to note is that the market creates *different* 'winners' and 'losers', the education market only working for those who can afford to operate in it. Commenting on the development of the education market in the United States, Moore and Davenport observe: 'Given the discretion exercised in recruitment, screening and selection, there was an overwhelming bias towards establishing procedures and standards at each step in the admissions procedure that screened out "problem" students and admitted the best students, with "best" being defined as students with good academic records, good attendance, good behaviour, a mastery of English, and no special learning problems' (Moore and Davenport, 1990, p. 201).

The losers in the education market will, like the losers under the public monopoly, have to accept the system whether they like it or not but, unlike the losers under the public monopoly, will be unable to avail themselves of any alternatives. For example, Green's vision for increased parental choice in the education market would mean LEAs providing a residual education for the children of the poor. That such provision, in inadequately resourced inner city 'sink' schools serving disadvantaged populations, would have to be inferior to make choice meaningful, appears to cause Green little concern.

Within the more limited 'quasi market' developed in Britain, increased competition between schools could, paradoxically, be counter-productive. First, rather than promoting diversity and innovation, educational quality and leadership may become diluted or compromised if schools and their owners/managers are required to focus more on marketing, public relations, financial enterprise and corporate management (Evetts, 1996). Fear of failure could result in schools employing conservative strategies aimed at survival and playing safe in seeking to attract large numbers of pupils and the funding which accompanies them (Woods et al., 1996). Power et al.'s (1996) research shows GM schools pursuing the 'easy' route to academic excellence, reverting to selection by ability: 'The market mechanism orients the public entre-preneur towards attracting the effective consumer and the value-adding client, and away from a concern with service towards a commitment to survival' (Ball, 1993, p. 8). Second, the overall effectiveness of the education system could be eroded since it may reduce motivation for cooperation between schools. Third, concerns for the 'caring' aspects of a school may be given less prominence compared with traditional academic issues and/or 'hard' curriculum areas such as technology (Woods et al., 1996). Concern about public image and pupil recruitment may encourage less flexibility and responsiveness to pupils experi-encing emotional difficulties or who are not achievement-oriented, with consequent adverse effects on attendance, achievement and behaviour (ACESW and NASWE, 1991). Those who do not fit into the new world of the education market are increasingly likely to find themselves 'categorised out of "normal" education' (Tomlinson, 1982, p. 6) and confined to increasingly ghettoised and under-resourced special provision (Heward and Lloyd-Smith, 1990) (see also chapters 8 and 9).

In reality the market analogy in education is limited. In the true market the dissatisfied customer will shop somewhere else next time. Consumers of education (or more accurately their parents) cannot as easily 'shop around' for their children's education as they can for the weekly groceries, given the potential disruptiveness of moving a child from one school to another.

The welfare implications of education reforms are that parents really cannot shop around when their child is a high-cost/high-risk/low achiever. Neither these parents nor their children are perceived as welcome consumers by schools pressurised to maximise their ratings in performance tables. Rather they become the major recipients of LEAs' welfare services. In the next chapter we consider in more detail the role of education welfare and social work services for children and families.

CHAPTER 4

Social work and schooling

Introduction

The interface between social work and the education system has traditionally been characterised by competing and contradictory services for children in trouble at home or school. They receive very different sorts of social work assistance depending upon whether they are referred to a social services department or an education welfare service. Although the Seebohm Report (DHSS, 1968) recommended that the two services be integrated, a recommendation subsequently endorsed by the Association of Directors of Social Services (ADSS, 1978), only a handful of local authorities attempted integration. The services in most local authorities drifted even further apart with many mutual antagonisms fuelled by competing instructions from the (then) DES and DHSS. For example, at the time the DHSS was preparing for integrated services under the Children Act 1989, the DES published a Circular on the future of the Education Welfare Service (DES, 1986b) which arrived at markedly different conclusions. This circular sought to distance education welfare from mainstream social work with children, taking a narrow view of school attendance problems which ignored the potential role of the service in dealing with a wide range of childhood disadvantage (for an overview, see Blyth and Milner, 1987b).

This legislative separatism reflects two quite distinct traditions in social work which distinguishes children's problems in families from their problems at school. The two-strand development of social work responses to children is a peculiarly British phenomenon, a survey of European attitudes to the role of the family showing that while other European countries consider the bringing up *and* educating of children to be important, the British see providing love and affection as the most important task for the family (Family Policy Studies Centre, 1994). This is an important distinction in that it explains why social services work with children and families has become the mainstream service with education welfare remaining a marginalised and relatively under-developed service.

The high value placed on the family's capacity to provide love and affection for children has led to social workers in social services departments locating children's problems predominantly within individual 'dysfunctional' families. This view is supported by psychological theorising about the importance of children developing secure attachments to their parents (see, for example, Bowlby, 1980) with interventions resulting from such assessments of this genesis of children's problems tending to be largely psychosocial whether the therapy is for individual children (see, for example, Fraiberg, 1988) or whole families (see, for example, Walrond-Skinner, 1976). There have been many criticisms of this somewhat restricted approach to social work with children. For example, Ahmad (1991) contends that it neglects issues such as identity or community and Ingleby (1984) maintains that it neglects the influence of social factors on family functioning, thus leading to a sort of psychological reductionism which places unreasonable expectations on mothers for the healthy development of their children and ignores the role of fathers in families (Milner, 1996). Additionally, Frones (1995) maintains that this focus on appropriate adult–child relationships for the psychic health of children neglects the influential role of child–child relationships on children's socialisation.

Within this tradition, a social worker in a children and families' social services department dealing with, say, a black child removed from an abusive family, would probably offer therapy which is based on meeting the child's emotional needs to do with affectional bonds. Despite information on the potentially damaging effects on such a child of being placed in a white foster home or having to change school, issues to do with race and education are unlikely to be prioritised. Although there has been a belated injunction from CCETSW emphasising the need for all social workers to acknowledge the importance of education in children's lives (CCETSW, 1995), the educational agenda for social workers employed in agencies such as social service departments is essentially one of neglect (Blyth and Milner, 1996c) with these not only being seen as the province of the education welfare service but also that service's workers being undervalued.

As we have shown in chapter 1, the education welfare service has historically located children's problems at school within a broader social framework of individual families' disadvantaged position in society, and much effort was deployed in attempting to ameliorate the impact of poverty. Although the general view of a society which values love and affection in families more highly than educational opportunity also devalues teachers' efforts, teachers have remained influential in the development of the education welfare service. Traditional perceptions of the education welfare officer as a 'handyman to the teacher' (Robinson, 1978) emphasising a coercive approach to interventions aimed at improving school attendance remain potent, although many teachers recognise the broader and more creative role social work may play within education.

This trend towards coercive interventions (the old image of the 'school bobby') is supported by a view of children *as* problems rather than children *with* problems. Peculiarly, while one branch of children's social work services can view a child with problems as a result of a dysfunctional family, there also exists the notion that children (and their families) are dangerous. Historically, children have always been perceived as a danger to society (for an overview, see Pearson, 1983) and children form convenient scapegoats for any moral panic, such as a concern about juvenile crime levels (see, for example, the Department for Education complaint that '(the) cycle of criminality is too often triggered by being truant from school' (DFE, 1992a, p. 6)).

The recurrent call to 'discipline' children by ensuring that they are in school and being educated in a way which will fit them to become 'good' citizens has been a constant pressure on the education welfare service to fulfil a controlling rather than a welfare function. Thus, interventions such as the Leeds adjournment scheme provided a veneer of legitimacy for overtly punitive and coercive measures to tackling non-attendance at school and bolstered the popular image of the education welfare officer as a 'school bobby'. This image is currently at risk of being revived under 'Truancy Watch' schemes, disillusion with welfare, and the explicit return to authoritarian regimes, such as one London borough's abandonment of 'softline' social work intervention in favour of the 'rottweiler approach' to non-attendance (Scott-Clark and Burke, 1996). (See also chapter 7.) Whether the child is seen as having problems or being a problem, both strands of social work services for children serve to deflect attention away from broader societal forces which impact seriously on child development.

As we have shown in chapters 1 and 2, while international conventions have made explicit the previously implicit right of children to education conferred by domestic education legislation, access to education and the opportunity to take full advantage of it are compromised by social factors and socio-economic adversity, even in a comparatively affluent society such as Britain.

Tasks of the education welfare service

Local education authorities have no legal obligation to provide an education welfare service nor to employ education welfare officers. Consequently the service has no inherent statutory remit. The lack of both a statutory basis and central government directions concerning the role of the service, other than stressing its role in relation to school attendance, are held by several commentators to be the major reasons for the wide variation to be found among different education welfare services throughout the country. While this can enable LEAs to respond flexibly to local priorities and need, it has been argued that: 'even allowing for . . . local differences, however, the practice of EWSs varies to an unacceptable degree' (DES, 1989b, pp. 30–1).

In practice there is general consensus that a central responsibility of the service is dealing with school attendance (DES, 1984, 1989a, b; Dunn, 1987; Halford, 1994; OFSTED, 1995b) although disputes about methods and styles of intervention remain (see chapter 7 for a fuller discussion).

In addition a focus on ensuring that 'children are able to benefit to

the full from whatever educational opportunities are offered them'
(DES, 1984) legitimates a much wider range of activities than simply
trying to get children into school. Various policy statements (e.g. DFE
and Welsh Office, 1992; DFE, 1994 b–e; DFE and DOH, 1994a) and
analyses of the role of education welfare services (DES, 1984, 1986b,
1989a, b; Dunn, 1987; Halford, 1994; Learmonth, 1995) indicate the
wide range of activities with which education welfare services
throughout the country are involved, although not every service would
claim to be involved with all of these: work with disabled children and
children with statements of 'special educational need'; child protection
work; monitoring and regulation of child employment; working with
pre-school age children (e.g. assisting parents to obtain nursery
placements); home–school liaison; inter-agency liaison; preventive
programmes on drugs (especially solvent abuse); working with children
exhibiting disruptive behaviour and/or at risk of exclusion from school;
securing alternative education provision for persistent non-attenders and
children excluded from school; providing individual and/or group work
for persistent non-attenders and/or parents; providing information/
advocacy/mediation for children excluded from school and their
parents; providing in-service training for other staff, including teachers;
preparing reports for courts; providing advice/administration concerning
welfare benefits; participation in the juvenile justice system; work with
pregnant schoolgirls/school-age mothers; work with 'young carers';
work with children and families on relationship difficulties and work
with traveller children.

The need for support on a wide range of 'welfare' issues is demonstrated by research conducted on behalf of the Association of Teachers
and Lecturers: 'In a climate of increasing social problems owing to the
interrelated factors of unemployment, increase in petty crime, drug
abuse and family breakdown, schools often provide the most readily
available and accessible source of counselling and information. Consequently many schools appear to have become an unfunded branch of the
social services' (Webb, 1994, p. 71), leading to a proposal that every
school should have its own social worker. However, the ability of social
services departments to provide such assistance is clearly circumscribed
by resource shortages and departmental priorities. The Audit Commission (1994) found that social services' child and family work was
largely focused on child protection. Similarly OFSTED noted that:
'involvement of the social services in schools was rare. In many local
authorities social workers were so pressurised that they dealt with
immediate urgent cases and priority concerns such as child protection'
(OFSTED, 1995a, p. 8).

While it has been suggested that some of the tasks in which
education welfare services are engaged may be 'peripheral' to the main
focus on school attendance, it is worth bearing in mind the functions
other than school attendance that the government itself has seen
appropriate to associate with education welfare. These include:
home–school liaison (DFE and DOH, 1994a); child protection (DES,

1988; DFEE, 1995a); 'special educational needs' (DFE, 1994b); drug abuse (DFE and Welsh Office, 1992); prevention of exclusions (DFE, 1994d; DFE and DOH, 1994a); planning and managing the return of a previously excluded pupil (DFE, 1994c, d); the integration of an excluded pupil into a new school (DFE, 1994d); work with individual children and families who may have particular emotional problems or relationship difficulties with their peers (DFE, 1994c); liaison between schools and pupils receiving home tuition (DFE, 1994e); dealing with 'particularly difficult pupils' through providing advice to school staff, chairing meetings involving school representatives and parents, and contributing to programmes of in-service training for teachers (DFE, 1994c).

Potentially the education welfare service has a major role in providing an essential service for children. However, not only has government failed to appreciate this and define the role more clearly but the haphazard resourcing of education welfare and its disproportionate level of exposure to cutbacks in local education authority budgets has meant that a consistent professional response has been difficult to develop.

Staffing and organisation of education welfare services

From a national study of education welfare agencies in England and Wales, Halford (1994) found a 1:4 ratio between managerial and fieldwork staff in education welfare agencies, although there were individual differences between LEAs and in some services, managers also undertook fieldwork tasks. However, further details are not provided and, since Halford's study did not investigate the provision of clerical and administrative support within education welfare services, the extent to which professional staff might be unproductively engaged on administrative or clerical tasks is not documented. This is clearly a factor which needs to be considered in determining the most effective use of resources.

Halford notes that little use appears to be made of volunteers, 13 services (11.8 per cent) using volunteers compared with 97 (88.2 per cent) which did not. While the use of volunteers is contentious in the context of potential budget cuts and consequent staff reductions, and effort is needed to recruit and support suitable volunteers, it is arguable that further consideration should be given to the possible use of volunteers by education welfare services as a means of enhancing the quality of provision.

Halford's research generally supports other sources concerning EWO:pupil ratios. This demonstrated ratios ranging from 1:719 to 1:10,035. If all EWO staff (including managers) are taken into account a national average EWO:pupil ratio is calculated at 1:2,443. However, the ratio reduces to 1:3,072 if fieldwork staff only are included. More recent but less comprehensive data have been provided by the National

Association of Social Workers in Education (NASWE, 1996), based on information from 59 LEAs in England and relating to the year 1993–4. This showed EWO:pupil ratios ranging from 1:1,350 (Liverpool) to 1:6,500 (Cheshire and Oldham). In evidence to the House of Commons Education Committee NASWE stated its position on staffing: 'It is this Association's view that in order to offer an effective professional service to ensure that children's interests are adequately safeguarded and effective preventative work carried out a ratio of 1:2,000 is recommended. However, in making a recommendation the Association is aware of the various roles an LEA expect an EWO/ESW to carry out on their behalf, some of which do not relate to school attendance and child employment and can place extra restraints on the workload on an EWO/ESW' (House of Commons, 1995, p. 128).

With regard to training and qualifications, Halford found that about a fifth of education welfare staff held a professional social work qualification. This in itself represented a thirty-fold increase compared with qualification levels recorded by MacMillan (1977), and 40 per cent of authorities seconded staff to Diploma in Social Work programmes. However, Halford also found that a fifth of services had no social work qualified staff at all, and very few authorities supported staff in obtaining further (post-qualifying/post-graduate) qualifications. Possession of a social work qualification is not a national requirement for employment as an education welfare officer, although a small number of LEAs require this for appointment, especially at senior levels, while many others regard it as a desirable qualification. Halford's survey also revealed that a large number of staff held other qualifications, e.g. first and post-graduate degrees, higher diplomas and 6.8 per cent held a teaching qualification. Given the poor response of social services social work staff to educational matters, it could be argued that the Diploma in Social Work is not necessarily the most appropriate qualification for education welfare officers but the lack of any agreed professional qualification means that education welfare officers are disadvantaged in both intra- and inter-agency work. Additionally, it contributes to their continuing marginalisation, preventing their voice being heard in debates about the form of child welfare delivery.

Towards an effective education welfare service

The OFSTED report *The Challenge for Education Welfare* (OFSTED, 1995b) indicates that the effectiveness of education welfare services is dependent on: the quality of support provided by the LEA; firm leadership by experienced senior managers; clarity and agreement about the aims and objectives of the service and appropriate training.

The debate about the range of duties and depth of work it is appropriate to expect of the education welfare service needs to take into account the following issues:

- docs the task need to be done at all?
- can the task be delegated to any other service or agency and what would be the implications of doing so?
- what are the implications of not doing particular tasks, especially in terms of local authorities' service pledges and legal responsibilities?

In order for the service to retain credibility with schools, pupils, their parents and other services, the LEA must ensure a reasonable balance between the remit and expectations of the service and the resources required to carry this out efficiently.

While the scope for work with individual families and with individual and groups of children remains, there is increasing recognition of the role education welfare officers/education social workers may play within the concept of a 'whole school approach' (as we have noted in chapter 2).

Inevitably the work undertaken by education welfare officers on behalf of individual pupils may bring them into conflict with schools. Where whole school approaches have not been fully institutionalised, some teachers may not recognise their own or the school's role (as opposed to factors external to the school) in promoting good attendance or behaviour. Another possible source of tension could arise where education welfare officers assist or advise parents in appealing against their child's exclusion from school. Government data (DFE, 1993) showed that, despite provisions for appeals and review of exclusions decisions, exclusions were rarely challenged by parents, local education authorities or school governing bodies, and where parents exercised their right of appeal against their child's exclusion their chances of success were slim indeed. At least some educationalists perceive parents' rights of appeal against exclusion as a threat to the maintenance of school discipline, rather than as a demonstration of appropriate checks and balances to the powers of head teachers.

Given the education welfare officer's role in promoting school attendance it is also worth highlighting a key relationship between monitoring school attendance and exclusion practices. In chapter 9 we review evidence concerning schools' use of informal and irregular means for excluding pupils. Since the education welfare officer is likely to be the only regular independent scrutineer of school attendance records, their investigation of absences may represent the only check against the use of such unlawful and unofficial exclusions.

The education welfare officer's traditional focus on individual pupils and the development of home–school links, and their freedom from the constraints of the school timetable, provide the opportunity to identify issues which need addressing within schools and on which all members of the school community can work. The education welfare officer can help ensure that pupils' individual learning needs are identified and appropriately targeted by the school thus preventing potential behaviour and/or attendance problems. Such intervention may take the form of group or individual work with the pupil. Alternatively, it may involve the education welfare officer advising on curricular issues, resulting in time-tabling or other structural changes. Education welfare officers can contribute to the further development of 'whole school' approaches through, for example:

* resisting the pressure to take exclusive responsibility for attendance issues;
* ensuring that initiatives to improve behaviour and attendance do not focus excessively on work with individual pupils perceived to be 'at risk', while ignoring the contribution of the curriculum and school processes;
* ensuring that school staff are aware of relevant 'out-of-school' factors;
* fostering links between the school and the community it serves;
* encouraging consistency within and between schools in the categorisation and recording of absence and policies and practice regarding pupil behaviour.

Elsewhere within the welfare network the concepts of 'partnership' and 'cooperation' across organisational and professional boundaries regarding services for children has received government support (e.g. DOH, 1991a; DFE, 1994 b–d; DFE and DOH, 1994a–c), albeit within a legislative and social policy context which promotes contrary developments such as 'internal markets' and competition. Legislative imperatives which broadly impose on health, education and welfare agencies a duty to cooperate (e.g. Children Act 1989 and Education Act 1993) are circumscribed so that a request for assistance may be refused if this is deemed unnecessary or inconsistent with other functions, or if the agency is able to plead insufficient resources. The cause of effective inter-agency cooperation is further hindered by increasing pressures on the budgets of local government agencies, including threats of financial penalties for overspending. It is hardly surprising, therefore, that contemporary commentators have found little evidence of effective cooperation within the welfare network (e.g. Blyth and Milner, 1990; Audit Commission and HMI, 1992; Audit Commission, 1994; Parsons *et al.*, 1994; OFSTED, 1995a, 1996b; SSI and OFSTED, 1995; National Commission of Inquiry into the Prevention of Child Abuse, 1996; SSI, 1996). Commenting on the relationship between education and social services Sinclair (1994) observes: 'there is evidence of a growing tension between professionals in education and Social Services Departments, often despite feelings of goodwill and shared aims, but the ability to work together effectively is being hampered by arguments over budgets and the growing practice of having to contract or buy in services once freely exchanged'.

Contemporary challenges for social work and schooling

The Children Act 1989, which came into force in 1990, provided a long-needed restructuring of child welfare services. It was influenced by the Cleveland Report (Secretary of State, 1988), a House of Commons Inquiry into children in local authority care (House of Commons, 1984) and Britain's endorsement of the UN Convention on the Rights of the Child. Unusually, the legislation enjoyed parliamentary support from all political parties and widespread support from all child care professionals. It was envisaged that the central tenet of the Act – the paramountcy of the welfare of the child – indicated that, finally, there was consensus about the value of children's rights and interest in their well-being which would remove many of the old tensions and contradictions in child-care legislation and welfare services, particularly as the Children Act was supported by the introduction of a Child Support Agency aimed at reducing the burden of lone-parent families on the state by tracking down maintenance-avoiding fathers and making more explicit their role in families.

However, consensus about the paramountcy of the welfare of the child very quickly proved untranslatable into practice. As Kadushin and Martin (1981) have pointed out, the concept is so bland that it can mean anything. In a recession-gripped country with a large number of elderly people who may become an additional burden on the state, an increasing number of non-child households, more women opting to remain childless or limiting family size (Jones, 1992), and considerable opposition on the part of fathers to the efforts of the Child Support Agency, it became clear that there was little meaningful commitment to child welfare. At the time the Children Act 1989 became law, children had become marginalised in a society which saw them as more of a current social cost than a social investment for the future (Leach, 1994). The effects on children's mental health have been severe, Rutter (1991b) arguing that there is evidence of a post-war increase in many forms of child psychiatric disorder which are influenced by prevailing social conditions. The NHS Health Advisory Service has itself indicated that up to 40 per cent of children – twice the number previously estimated – were at risk of suffering some form of mental illness (Kennedy, 1996).

In summary, the challenges and difficulties for social work in education are ones in which services have to be provided in a context in which children are not regarded positively although their parents are scrutinised for possible abuse; the Department of Health and Department of Education and Employment appear to lack a coordinated approach to child welfare which also leads to budgetary competition; and there is serious underfunding in all branches of child-care services with a tendency to rely on short-term project funding which has little impact on broad trends. Despite these difficulties, the task for social workers in child-welfare organisations has become much bigger but the emphasis remains on child protection issues, with no real commitment to child welfare, this being true for children both in and out of public care.

In order to move forward, social work needs to address the very real problem of defining the role of the modern education welfare officer and begin to coordinate the separate services. The task, as we say, is a large and daunting one but in subsequent chapters we outline in detail the main areas where pupils experience problems. We suggest that an understanding of these problem areas is one for all social workers, whatever their agency context.

CHAPTER 5

The education of children in public care

Introduction

There are two major strands to the relationship between education and public care. Most significantly, since the middle of the 1970s there has been mounting evidence indicating serious deficiencies in the quality of both the educational experiences of children in care in Britain and their educational attainment. However, nearly two decades after such inform- ation was generally available little evidence existed of its impact on policy and practice: 'The education of children in care is not subject to negligence; it is largely a non-issue because so often it is not seen as significant in terms of the confirmation of the individual or the part it can play in compensating for, or subsuming (rather than repairing), "damage"' (Fletcher-Campbell and Hall, 1990, p. 104). Second, evi- dence is emerging of the importance of educational factors in precipi- tating admission to care and affecting care placements. For example, Bennathan (1992) and Cohen and Hughes (1994) suggest that exclusion from school may increase the risk of children coming into care. Jackson and Cairns (1986) also note that foster placement breakdown may be prompted by difficulties the child is facing at school. In a study of children who were assessed for social services provision in a London borough, Sinclair *et al.* (1993) note that education was a 'hugely significant' factor behind the request for local authority services, 'persistent non-school attendance' identified by both social workers and parents as the main presenting problem in two thirds of the cases.

Much of the available substantive research evidence is based on the experiences of children who were at school and in care during the 1960s, 70s and 80s, i.e. before the major legislative and policy changes affecting both the British education and child care systems in the 1980s and 1990s. Some caution needs to be exercised, therefore, in applying evidence from the past to the present. However, it would also be a mistake to assume that the mere passage of time had changed the situation so dramatically for children in public care, or to pretend that rhetoric necessarily reflects accepted practice. Past neglect of the education of children in public care reflected official views such as those expressed by a 'senior government official' to a former children's officer: 'It is no part of your job to try to provide for a child better than his own parents would have done' (cited in Jackson, 1989, p. 138). However, there is less evidence that contemporary practice reflects the fundamental ideological shift expressed by the Utting Committee that: 'Care authorities should act to remedy the educational disadvantage of children in their care, and do all that a good parent would do to ensure that children's needs are met' (DOH, 1991a, p. 10).

There is now a volume of undisputed evidence that children in public care perform poorly on objective measures of academic attainment. They exhibit comparatively high levels of disturbed behaviour in school and are more likely to be absent or excluded from school. Their longer-term employment prospects remain poor. (For a fuller discussion see, for example, Essen et al., 1976; Stein and Carey, 1983; Stein, 1986, 1994; Parker, 1988; Heath et al., 1989, 1994; Fletcher-Campbell and Hall, 1990; Biehal et al., 1992; Firth, 1992, 1995; Audit Commission, 1994; Cheung and Heath, 1994; Colton and Heath, 1994; SSI and OFSTED, 1995; Stirling, 1996.) Stein (1994) notes that the low level of edu- cational attainment of care leavers leaves them 'ill-prepared to compete in an increasingly competitive and shrinking youth labour market' (Stein, 1994, p. 354).

Quality of education provided for children in care

Firth (1992) comments that there is an assumption that children in the care system have the weight of the local authority behind them to secure their rights to educational equality and opportunity. Evidence that this is patently not the case in many instances first surfaced following publication in 1976 of the analysis of data from the National Child Development Study (based on a study of people born in Britain during one week in 1958 which provides a longitudinal analysis of the impact, particularly on health, education and employment, of changing econ- omic and social conditions and policies). Information about the study cohort at ages seven and eleven years provided clear evidence that children in public care suffered poorer educational experiences than their peers who had not been in care (Essen et al., 1976). However, the authors were unable to determine whether the care group's low edu- cational attainment could be attributed to their pre-care experiences (most having lived in disadvantaged circumstances) or to the care experience itself. In chapter 1 we briefly reviewed the Leeds adjourn- ment scheme, indicating that this provided no evidence that committal to local authority care improved the education of children who were previously not attending school. In another research study Carlen (1987) notes that the criminal careers of a group of young women could be traced to their committal to care for non-attendance at school.

Fletcher-Campbell and Hall (1990) report on an eighteen-month study focusing on provision for the educational needs of children in care. Information was sought by questionnaire from all Social Services Departments in England and Wales. This was supplemented with details of all children of statutory school age who had been in care for more than six months in three authorities and a more detailed study of twenty individual children was also undertaken. Fifty-five (47 per cent) of the 117 Social Services Departments approached replied, although only 43 (37 per cent) provided the information requested. The survey of children reveals that a significant group of children in care experience a stable educational placement, associated with a secure and long-term period in care. However, two thirds had experienced educational problems and had had changes of school. Only a third attended mainstream school. Nearly a quarter had truanted and for a significant proportion truancy was either a regular occurrence or sustained over a period of time. More than a third of the children in care had experienced changes of school for reasons other than normal transfer. Fourteen per cent had attended three or more schools. For more than two thirds of the children the reasons for the changes were essentially care-related, e.g. change of care placement, temporary or assessment placements, or for issues relating to the care placement. About a quarter of the changes were due to problems related to school or change following assessment for 'special educational needs'. Over half the children had significant problems at school or had 'special educational needs'. Fletcher-Campbell and Hall conclude that, on the basis of their educational experiences, children in care are not an homogeneous group and that six distinct groups could be identified according to their educational experience:

- children who had no identified problems or change of school (135 children – 34%);
- children who had no problems but had had changes of school since entering care for reasons other than routine school transfer (41 children – 10%);
- children who had significant problems in school (45 children – 11%);
- children who were subject of a statement of 'special educational need' but had 'stable placements' and no other problems with school (53 children – 13%);
- children who had truanted but had no other problems with school (43 children – 11%);
- children with a combination of problems and who had faced severe disruption to their education (82 children – 21%).

In 1995 the Social Services Inspectorate and OFSTED reported on a joint inspection of education for 'looked-after' children conducted in four local authority areas (SSI and OFSTED, 1995). The inspectors found that the educational achievement of children was low, particularly for secondary school age children. None of these children's teachers thought them likely to achieve five subjects at Grade A–C in GCSE, compared to the general school population where 38.3 per cent of Year 11 pupils in maintained secondary schools achieved five or more subjects at grade A–C in 1993. Approximately 12 per cent of the looked-after children were not in school either because of non-attendance or exclusion, although there were wide variations between the four local authorities.

These findings reflect an earlier report from the Audit Commission (1994) which showed that while 56 per cent of 'looked-after' children attended school, and a further 10 per cent were being educated in social services units, just over a third were not attending school. Of these over 40 per cent were permanently, indefinitely or temporarily excluded; 39 per cent were 'refusing to attend' and 7 per cent had no school place. In one local authority 40 per cent of five- to sixteen-year olds in children's homes were receiving no education. The SSI/OFSTED report concludes: 'The care and education services in general are failing to promote the educational achievement of children who are looked after. The standards which children achieve are too low and often the modest progress they make in primary schools is lost as they proceed through the system. Despite the clear identification of this problem in several research studies and by committees of enquiry, little has been done in practice to boost achievement' (SSI and OFSTED, 1995, p. 41).

Consumer views

Relatively few studies have sought to ask directly care recipients about their educational experiences. Notable exceptions are 'leaving care' studies (Stein and Carey, 1983; Stein, 1986; Biehal *et al.*, 1992) and a survey of over six hundred young people in residential care and foster care conducted by the Who Cares? Trust and the National Consumer Council (Fletcher, 1993). Stein (1994) notes that in the 'Leaving Care' study nearly all the young people interviewed reported that at school they felt their care status made them different, the 'odd one out', the subject of curiosity, of teasing and even abuse.

Fletcher's study reveals some 'stark contrasts' in the young people's experiences of education. Some recounted positive experiences of motivation and educational attainment, support and encouragement by residential and foster carers, while others recalled 'deeply disturbing experiences' of teasing, bullying, stigma, frequent disruptions, delays in securing a school placement following placement moves, poor conditions for study, distractions, non-attendance and low expectations by both teachers and carers. Those who reported an improvement in their education while in care 'almost exclusively' associated this with being supported, encouraged and settled, and in some cases because the difficulties which had led to them being 'looked after' had improved.

Educational outcomes, foster and residential care

The literature indicates that there are particular factors associated with residential care which might pose barriers to children's educational progress. Fletcher's (1993) survey highlights a range of negative features associated with being in residential care: being in more trouble at school, peer-group pressure not to attend school, prolonged absence from school, low expectations of school attendance and little encouragement from staff.

Other evidence suggests that residential social workers' own limited educational experiences may result in their low educational aspirations for the young people in their care (e.g. Parker, 1988; Stein, 1994). The low school attainments of residential social work staff was also highlighted by Millham *et al.* (1980). Only 32 per cent reported enjoying their own schooldays; 62 per cent of those who had taken the 'eleven plus' examination had failed it and 59 per cent had left school by age sixteen with 'mediocre' attainments. Since this study was largely based on staff with management responsibilities who had been seconded to a training course, the educational experience of less senior staff may be even less auspicious. Possible implications of this are that residential staff may be less likely to make demands on either schools or children and may not expect the children in their care to have any greater academic success than they had achieved themselves.

Characteristic conditions and the style of life in residential homes may present further barriers. A residential unit may offer limited or no privacy for the completion of homework and study, and routinely high turnover of both staff and children means that residents are rarely able to develop a relationship with a member of staff who is in a position to take a long-term active interest in the child's educational experience. (We discuss the implications of placement 'turnover' in more detail below.)

While all children in public care run the risk of being stigmatised by other young people and adults, those in residential care may be particularly exposed to negative attitudes. Carlen *et al.* (1992) cite one residential worker: 'A number of schools are prejudiced against children in care and respond to even the slightest misdemeanour by asking the care staff to remove them from school. Frequently they refuse to have them back' (Carlen *et al.*, 1992, p. 87).

Although clear distinctions in the effects of foster and residential care may be difficult to establish because many children in public care have experience of both, the limited data available suggest that, while still providing cause for concern, children and young people in foster care fare less badly educationally than their counterparts in residential care.

Fletcher-Campbell and Hall (1990) observe that children in foster care are less likely to experience exclusion from school. Respondents to Fletcher's (1993) enquiry who had experienced foster care were more likely than those in residential care to consider their education had improved as a result of being in care (43 per cent compared to 32 per cent), while 17 per cent of those in foster care and 38 per cent in residential care considered that their schooling had deteriorated as a result of being in care and 40 per cent of those in foster care and 30 per cent in residential care thought there had been no change.

Reporting on the findings of a longitudinal study of the educational progress and behaviour of a group of 49 children aged between eight and fourteen in long-term foster care, Colton and Heath (1994) and

Heath *et al.* (1989, 1994) note their relative disadvantage when compared with a similar group of children whose families were in receipt of social work assistance but who remained with their families. As might be expected, foster children exhibiting major behavioural problems were also poor achievers academically. However, foster children who had no significant behavioural problems also scored below the national average on standardised measures of educational attainment and showed no sign of relative improvement over the period of the study. Despite their ostensibly favourable circumstances (most were in long-term settled placements with foster parents who were able to provide an environment conducive to educational progress) foster children experienced comparable educational disadvantage to other children who have experienced local authority care. The implications of these findings are that conventional explanations for the low educational attainment of children in care, such as the particular difficulties of residential care, insecure or impermanent placements or frequent placement changes (see below for further discussion of these) do not fully explain the differences in outcome.

Social services' education provision

While the majority of 'looked-after' children are educated in local authority mainstream or 'special' schools, education for a minority may be provided by social services departments themselves. Past reviews of such education provision have been uniformly negative (e.g. DES, 1978; DHSS, 1981) a trend maintained in a 1992 survey conducted by the DES in which 28 education units run by 23 Social Services Departments were inspected (DES, 1992). While the report cites evidence of some effective and imaginative work, there were wide discrepancies in standards between institutions. The units, which were predominantly small, found it difficult to provide a balanced curriculum. 'Serious defects' in accommodation constrained the curriculum in fifteen establishments, while in sixteen the curriculum had 'significant deficiencies' of breadth and balance. Teaching and care teams tended to 'work separately with no commonly considered rationale'. The inspectors were concerned that acknowledgement of pupils' difficulties might result in low expectations about their educational achievements, and that attending to their particular personal and social needs could restrict their access to a 'broad and balanced' education. Similar curricular limitations in such units have also been noted by Fletcher-Campbell and Hall (1990) and SSI and OFSTED (1995).

Education and employment prospects of care recipients

Cheung's and Heath's (1994) analysis of National Child Development Study data confirms the continuing educational and occupational disadvantage experienced by those who have been in care, but also that formal educational qualifications and employment prospects varied according to the nature of the care experience. Although, like previous researchers, they were unable to pinpoint the precise causes of this, they comment that long-term care had done little to off-set the legacy of any difficulties which existed prior to the child's admission to care. Rather than basing their analysis of the data on simplistic 'in care' and 'never in care' classifications, however, Cheung and Heath isolated five sub-categories of care status, according to the child's age at entry into care and the length of time spent in care. Children who had experienced short periods of care before the age of one year enjoyed average educational and occupational outcomes. All of those who had left care at later ages had educational attainments significantly below the national average for their peers who had never been in care. However, given their formal academic attainments, most of these fared no worse occupationally than their similarly qualified peers who had never been in care. The most disadvantaged young people were those who entered care at or before the age of eleven and did not leave care until after eleven, who had even lower occupational attainments than would have been expected on the basis of their qualifications. Variations in care experience and occupational outcomes were also noted by Biehal *et al.* (1992) – 48 per cent of those leaving Community Homes with Education and 65 per cent of those leaving independence units were subsequently unemployed. While the research does not provide explanations for these outcomes, Stein (1994) speculates that these young people may have already been the most disadvantaged at the point of admission to care which itself could have added to their educational difficulties through the fragmentation and weakening of family and neighbourhood ties.

Movements in care and educational outcomes

As indicated earlier, placement changes have been cited as a potential source of educational difficulties for young people in care. Multiple placement and consequent disruption to education is a common experience for young people in care (e.g. Stein and Carey, 1983; Berridge, 1985; Millham *et al.*, 1986; Stein, 1986; Berridge and Cleaver, 1987; Biehal *et al.*, 1992) although more likely to affect those in residential care (Fletcher-Campbell and Hall, 1990). Berridge (1985) reports that several children in his study could not remember how many schools they had attended. Firth (1995), in a study of over 200 young people in local authority care, notes a correlation between frequency of placement move and the risk of permanent exclusion from school. Eight out of nine young people experiencing five or more changes in place-ment were permanently excluded. However, the small number of children experiencing frequent placement moves and the possibility that both disruption to school and care placements may be related to the child's behaviour mean that it would be premature to infer a causal relationship between frequency of placement change and the likelihood of exclusion from school.

Generally, the longer a child is in care the more likely they are to experience placement change. Eighty-four per cent of those who stay in care for two years or more move placement at least once and 56 per cent move two or more times (Bullock *et al.*, 1993). A young person's care experience may include periods of being in and out of care and care placements may include both foster and residential care.

Stein (1994), reporting on the 'leaving care' studies, comments on the association between movement in care and poor educational attainment and the fact that the majority of young people in these studies experience frequent moves. In the *Prepared for Living?* study only 9 per cent of the sample remained in the same placement throughout their time in care and three quarters of those who had experienced four or more moves in care had no qualifications compared to only half of those who had made no moves. In *Leaving Care* just over three quarters of young people had experienced three or more placements in care and just over 40 per cent five or more placements, or an average of 4.4 per person. In *Living Out of Care* over half the young people had between seven and twelve placements by the time they were sixteen years of age and the average for the sample was six placements per young person. Fletcher-Campbell and Hall (1990) report a smaller proportion of young people experiencing multiple placements and indicate that placement change does not invariably result in a change of school. In addition, they observe that disruption to education placement is differentially experienced by different groups of young people.

Stein (1994) comments that the bare statistics might fail to convey the nature and impact of repeated placement disruptions. Since a high proportion of the young people had entered care as teenagers the placement moves were compressed into a relatively short time period: 'Education as a developmental process is therefore likely to have little meaning given the disruption to syllabuses, course work and examination preparation' (Stein, 1994, p. 353).

The vast majority of children and young people who enter local authority care return home. The educational implications of a child returning home from care may be similar to those associated with a change of placement in care. Bullock *et al.* (1994) note that social workers showed very little interest in the academic achievement of young people returning home after an extensive period in care. Rather they were content if the children merely went to school and behaved satisfactorily. Compared to other long-term absentees, however (e.g. pregnant girls and children who had been hospitalised or had long-term illness), the return to school of those who had been in care for over a year was especially problematic. School and home problems were more often than not mutually reinforcing, possibly involving peer-relationship difficulties, attainment and attendance difficulties, abuse and delinquency. The researchers also report that return to school was no more likely to be considered as part of the return strategy than any other move in care. In many instances, therefore, schools were unprepared for the child's return. Similarly, Fletcher-Campbell and Hall (1990) note instances of children returning from out-of-authority placements with inadequate notice of their return being given to the LEA, causing delay in providing a school place for them.

Bullock *et al.* (1994) comment that once the children had returned, teachers appeared to find difficulty in conceptualising return to school as a problem for the children. Often there was little awareness of the child having a 'social' career or that problems in one area could compound those in another. In addition, teachers made few attempts to build on the child's experiences while in care.

Social work perspectives

Fletcher-Campbell's and Hall's (1990) comment about the education of children in care as a non-issue encapsulates the conclusions reached by the majority of researchers about social work attitudes, practice and policy concerning the educational experiences of children in public care. The Department for Education and Department of Health note that: 'Children and young people being looked after, especially the older ones, are entitled to take part as far as possible in decisions that affect their lives and at least to have their views taken into account. Many children feel that they are not meaningfully involved in the decisions being taken about them, including those relating to moves of home or school' (DFE and DOH, 1994b, p. 9). Although this pronouncement accurately reflects (un)professional practice and we endorse fully the government's sentiments, we have previously commented on the irony that few other children are afforded any right of consultation over their education (Blyth and Milner, 1996c).

Consistently social workers have demonstrated more concern about the child's placement and emotional needs than their educational needs, despite evidence that attendance at an effective school can be crucial to a child's development (see chapter 2). As a result there is little evidence in social services departments of effective setting of education targets for young people in care, characterised by lack of involvement of teachers in planning and review procedures (SSI and OFSTED, 1995). Education issues are given very much second place and low priority is given by social services social workers to education when organising moves (e.g. Stein and Carey, 1983; Kahan, 1985; Jackson, 1987, 1988–9; Heath *et al.*, 1989, 1994; Bullock *et al.*, 1993, 1994). Schools often experience children arriving without advance information or any preparation, and frequently have to rely on fragmented information (SSI and OFSTED, 1995).

Responses by local authorities to Fletcher-Campbell's and Hall's enquiry (remembering that only just over a third of all local authorities provided any information at all) indicate that only a quarter identified educational stability and continuity as a priority for children in care.

Education was only one factor among many for the remainder for whom placement availability would take precedence over other considerations however desirable. This suggests that little has changed from earlier studies of decision making in child care. Melotte (1979) found that education was totally ignored by social workers and their managers in placement decisions for children entering care. In a study of social workers' objectives in child care planning only 16 out of 285 explicit objectives related to education. And even though half the children involved in the study were assessed as having school-related problems, for only six was educational improvement identified as a specific objective (Knapp *et al.*, 1985).

Even though social workers may claim concern about the personal development and long-term future of children in care, many demonstrate no awareness of how education and schooling might contribute to this. This may manifest itself in a variety of ways. First, the basis on which social workers judge the suitability of a school for young people in their care is more likely to be non-educational (i.e. in terms of its ability to cope with 'difficult' young people and be sympathetic and flexible) rather than on the school's academic record. Second, social workers may have little or no knowledge about the educational progress of children in care. Consequently, Fletcher-Campbell and Hall (1990) found that few social workers were aware whether the young person's educational potential was being fulfilled. In the SSI/OFSTED survey, for example, for 12 per cent of the total number of children (144) no information was given about their 'special educational needs' (ranging from 0.8 per cent (two) in one local authority to 19.4 per cent (85) in another. In *Prepared for Living?* (Biehal *et al.*, 1992) 19.5 per cent of social workers did not know whether the young people for whom they were responsible had any educational qualifications. Third, social workers may have low expectations of the educational potential of children in care. Jackson observes that local authority social workers: 'were critical of the "Looking After Children" scheme for setting excessively high standards and thus giving children a sense of failure. . . . Some social workers consider it unfair to give looked-after children educational advantages that poor parents looking after their own children are not able to give' (Jackson, 1994, p. 277). Fourth, social workers may place few demands on schools. Fletcher-Campbell and Hall observe that social services departments would not take on education as 'real parents' because 'we're all fellow employees' (Fletcher-Campbell and Hall, 1990, p. 40). Similarly, SSI and OFSTED identify a general reservation in social services to press for appeal in respect of exclusion from school: 'because of the likelihood of the harmful effects on relationships with schools. Appeals were viewed as a criticism rather than an opportunity to coolly discuss the events leading up to exclusion, to enable the child to understand the reasons for exclusion more clearly and for the school to reconsider the decisions in the light of any additional information' (SSI and OFSTED, 1995, p. 39).

Educational factors

As the Who Cares? Trust and National Consumer Council Survey (Fletcher, 1993) show, negative and humiliating treatment by teachers and other pupils are experienced by a number of young people in care. Aware of the potential for this, the Department for Education and Department of Health jointly called on teachers to challenge such discrimination (DFE and DOH, 1994b). Rather than outright hostility, though, indifference and ignorance appear to be more characteristic of school experiences. Part and parcel of this is the lack of knowledge which school staff have about individual children and, more generally about social services practices and procedures. Consequently the contribution which schools make to care planning and reviews for individual children tends to be poorly defined and, therefore, limited (SSI and OFSTED, 1995). At a practical level, there may well be problems for schools in teachers taking part in meetings, especially if schools have to resource teacher involvement – an inevitable consequence of LMS.

If schools receive little information from social workers about a 'looked-after' child they are unlikely to be better informed by the child's previous school: 'Commonly . . . school records were too disorganised to give a full account of the child to the next school or a new teacher' (SSI and OFSTED, 1995, p. 18).

Low expectations, not infrequently masked by more obvious welfare concerns that too much should not be expected from children and young people who already have considerably disadvantaged backgrounds, are more likely (Bullock *et al.*, 1993; Stein, 1994; see also chapter 2). Fletcher-Campbell and Hall (1990) note that young people themselves often criticise teachers for being too ready to excuse poor behaviour or work. Heath *et al.* (1989, 1994), though, are sceptical about the cause-effect relationship between teachers' low expectations and the poor educational progress of young people in care. Rather, they suggest that teachers' judgements are consequences rather than the causes of pupil performance.

The way forward

We have already commented on the tensions between education and child-care legislation and the consequences of these (see also chapter 3). As we have stated there, despite government exhortation to the contrary, the legislative framework hardly augurs well for coordination and cooperation at policy and practice levels. Unsurprisingly, therefore, there is little evidence of this regarding the education of children in public care. Where effective inter-agency cooperation does exist it is likely to rely on the efforts of committed individuals rather than established procedures (Fletcher-Campbell and Hall, 1990).

The Audit Commission (1994), SSI and OFSTED (1995) and OFSTED (1996b) highlight the characteristic failure of coordination between schools, education and social services departments. The OFSTED report on exclusions (OFSTED, 1996b) concludes that support strategies for 'looked-after' children in school remain inadequate because of the failure of effective liaison between social services, schools and LEAs. Walker (1994) notes that there is frequently a mis-match between education and social services' time-scales, work patterns and bureaucracies which militate against the right kind of intervention being delivered at the right time. Fletcher-Campbell and Hall (1990) identify the contrasting – and potentially conflicting – policy agenda of social services (favouring 'minimal intervention') and education (schools being more likely to think in terms of 'early warning').

Both the Parents' Charter (DES, 1991a; DFE, 1994a) and the Children Act 1989, promote the concept of parents as partners. The importance of the maintenance of parental contact for the educational achievement of young people in care is noted in Jackson's 'Successful in Care' study (Jackson, 1994). Commenting on the evaluation of the Department of Health 'Looking After Children' project (Parker *et al.*, 1991) Jackson also indicates that parents of all social classes give education much higher priority than most social workers, confirming the view that the local authority itself does not make a particularly responsible parent.

Despite rhetoric and exhortation there appears to be little evidence of the development of partnerships with parents of 'looked-after' children. The SSI/OFSTED report concludes that social services pay insufficient attention to involving those with parental responsibility and schools 'rarely understood' the importance of maintaining contact with those with parental responsibility. Consequently they were unlikely to keep those with parental responsibility informed of the child's school progress or of relevant school events (e.g. parents' evenings). There was little understanding of how to encourage parental interest in the child's education, reinforcing the parents' detachment from their child's life and progress.

For children and young people in local authority care 'school can provide one element of stability, continuity and belonging in an otherwise disrupted life' (Bullock *et al.*, 1994, p. 307). However, it is clear from the weight of evidence presented in this chapter that any report on the achievement of educators and care providers alike would include the admonition 'could do better . . . must try harder'.

The shortcomings in policy and practice and the fragmentation of parental responsibility for young people in public care have made inevitable the plethora of guidance and advice to local authorities, schools, residential homes and individual professionals and carers which are available from government bodies (DOH, 1991a; Audit Commission, 1994; DFE and DOH, 1994b; SSI and OFSTED, 1995; OFSTED, 1996b); interest groups (Fletcher, 1993); individual researchers (Jackson, 1988–9, 1995; Fletcher-Campbell and Hall, 1990; Stein, 1994) and other professionals (e.g. Levy and Kahan, 1991;

McParlin, 1996). In addition a number of local authorities have developed policy frameworks and dedicated services to promote improved service delivery (e.g. Walker, 1994; Firth, 1995).

The government and its agents clearly believe that they have established an appropriate legislative framework to encourage effective inter-agency collaboration and cooperation. As we have indicated in chapter 3, we, and others, do not share this conviction. Bullock *et al.* (1993) predict that increased autonomy of schools may further dis-advantage young people returning from care as they are unlikely to be among the 'star' pupils who will enhance the school's performance. Neither are their parents among those who are most likely to exercise their 'rights' in respect of their children's education. They also note that, despite the introduction of the National Curriculum, children moving schools may also be penalised by variations between different schools in the content and order of National Curriculum delivery.

Nevertheless we consider there is scope within existing legislative prescriptions and the policy implications which derive from them for improvements in practice.

Essentially a substantial shift in attitudes is required among those who organise or provide care or education for young people in the care system to recognise the importance of their educational needs and both the short- and long-term contribution that positive educational experiences and achievement can make to their lives. *Put simply, the local authority, acting as corporate parent, needs to take its responsibilities considerably more seriously.*

Fletcher-Campbell and Hall (1990) suggest that the promotion of equal educational opportunities for young people in care should focus on outcomes of, rather than merely access to, education. Such a prioritising of education is explicit in the codes developed by Jackson (1988–9); Fletcher-Campbell and Hall (1990); Fletcher (1993); DFE and DOH (1994b); Firth (1995); SSI and OFSTED (1995). Attitudinal and behavioural change encompasses social workers, carers and teachers resisting negative stereotyping of young people in care, maximising their education opportunities and challenging 'the non-achieving welfare culture of many existing children's homes dominated by low expectations' (Stein, 1994, p. 358).

This is not to ignore the question of resources. Appointing a member of staff in a residential establishment to take oversight of educational matters (Jackson, 1988–9); making primary school heads or secondary school pastoral staff responsible for 'looked-after' young people (DFE and DOH, 1994b); placing responsibility for the education of 'looked-after' young people on a senior manager in social services (DOH, 1991a; Levy and Kahan, 1991); providing adequate space in residential homes for homework and encouraging homework to be done, all have resource considerations. Arguably, though, these are issues of investing resources rather than simply spending them. A considerable amount of professional workers' time is already spent on what Parsons and his colleagues have described as 'debris management' (Parsons *et al.*,

1994), i.e. having to deploy resources as a consequence of decisions made and actions taken by others in the system or through someone not doing their job properly. Examples of 'debris management' include residential care staff who have to be employed for additional hours to care for young people excluded from school, as well as less easily quantifiable resource commitments of teachers, carers, social workers and others in dealing with the consequences of individual youngsters' disaffection and alienation, including placement breakdown. More positively, other work with young people in care and their families is likely to be more effective if the young person's educational needs are recognised and met. Jackson recounts the observations of a comprehensive school year head on the appointment of a member of staff in one children's home to take responsibility for residents' education: 'It's been the saving of the children; it's made all the difference. Before that they'd have stomach aches, headaches, anything rather than go to school, because they hadn't done their homework' (Jackson, 1988–9, p. 346).

CHAPTER 6

Children who care for others

Introduction

Awareness of 'young carers' – young people whose lives may be significantly affected by participating in the care of a sick or disabled family member – has expanded since the 1980s. Sources of evidence about young carers derive primarily from work in local areas (e.g. O'Neill, 1988; Page, 1988; Sandwell Caring for Carers Project, 1989; McCalman, 1990; Bilsborrow, 1992; Elliott, 1992; O'Neill and Platt, 1992; Wood, 1992; Aldridge and Becker, 1993, 1994; Blyth *et al.*, 1995; London Borough of Enfield, 1995); a national overview of young carers' projects (Dearden and Becker, 1995), and promotional work undertaken by the Carers' National Association with support from the Department of Health. To this have been added descriptions and evaluations of embryonic services for young carers in specific locations (Mahon and Higgins, 1995; Blyth *et al.*, 1996; Dearden and Becker, 1996; SSI, 1996). The efforts of activities over a relatively short period have been significant, young carers seen as a focus of Department of Health interest (Bowis, 1995; SSI, 1995a, b) and their need for services recognised in both child care (Children Act, 1989) and carers' legislation (Carers (Recognition and Services) Act, 1995). By 1996, 55 – approximately half of the total – English local authorities had produced policy documents regarding young carers (SSI, 1996).

Defining and identifying young carers

The difficulty in ascertaining the identity and number of young carers has been ascribed to: professionals' lack of awareness – including false assumptions about the availability and quality of family support; carers tending to regard themselves not as 'carers' but simply doing the 'responsible and obvious thing under the circumstances'; parents not wishing to be seen as 'failing' parents; parents' and young people's fears of negative consequences of identification (especially fear of separation and removal of one or more family member); and reluctance to talk to strangers about intimate tasks which may be carried out.

A central factor is the lack of a consistent definition of 'young carer'. The creation and application of different definitions of young carer in different studies mean that comparisons, especially regarding incidence, are impossible to make. Definitions vary according to the significance accorded to the nature and level of the tasks being undertaken, the impact of caring, and the person for whom care is being provided. The Department of Health Social Services Inspectorate has proposed a 'working' definition of a young carer as: 'a child or young person who is carrying out significant caring tasks and assuming a level of responsibility for another person, which would usually be taken by an adult. The term refers to children or young people under eighteen years caring for adults (usually their parents) or occasionally siblings. It does not refer to young people under eighteen years caring for their own children. Nor does the term refer to those children who accept an age appropriate role in taking increasing responsibility for household tasks in homes with a disabled, sick or mentally ill parent' (SSI, 1995a).

The focus on 'significant caring tasks', 'primary' caring (CNA, 1992) and Olsen's (1996) concept of 'heavily involved young carers', has the merit of potentially facilitating some quantitative measurement of the caring role. However, it does little to illuminate the *impact* of caring, which may have very little to do with the performance of specific tasks, the frequency with which they are carried out, or the time spent doing them. While knowledge of the tasks performed by young carers is undeniably important in terms of ascertaining entitlement to support and assistance, it is increasingly apparent that a more meaningful, if less easily quantifiable, approach is one which also takes account of the carer's subjective experience of caring and the impact of caring on their lives (Aldridge and Becker, 1993).

Highlighting the impact of caring on the young person's lifestyle, experiences and childhood raises further questions. In particular how should services respond to the needs of children and young people not fitting the prescribed definition of 'young carer' – such as, for example, those affected by the psychological and emotional distress caused by a parent suffering mental illness or a life-threatening illness (but who may not be undertaking recognised caring tasks), and those whose lifestyle, experiences and childhood are affected by caring responsibilities through family circumstances other than those resulting from illness or disability? Teachers, in particular, have expressed concern about the impact of domestic 'caring' responsibilities on the lives of such youngsters, who receive no support yet fall outside the 'young carers' remit and who receive no support (e.g. Sandwell Caring for Carers Project, 1989; London Borough of Enfield, 1995). Olsen (1996) also expresses concern that 'young carers' have been singled out for attention to the exclusion of other youngsters who may be involved in caring tasks or domestic labour. As we noted in chapter 1 the education of girls, in particular, has been constrained throughout history by their domestic responsibilities.

In this context two major methods have been employed to ascertain the incidence of young carers. First, initiatives and projects focused on young carers have sought basic quantitative data from targeted professional groups to provide approximate estimates. On the basis of the numbers of young carers identified in the Tameside and Sandwell studies, the Carers National Association estimated that at least 10,000 children nationally have 'primary' caring responsibilities (Carers National Association, 1993), a figure which has achieved national currency. Mahon and Higgins (1995), extrapolating from project data, consider that nationally there may be between 15,000 and 40,000 young carers. While they surmise this is probably an underestimate, Olsen (1996), who is sceptical of the extent of caring provided by children and young people, disagrees, asserting that it is more likely to be an over-estimate of the numbers of 'heavily involved young carers'. Second, attempts have been made to interrogate census and local and national data which provide information about family composition and the prevalence of illness and disability. Parker's analysis of data from the 1985 General Household Survey shows that 17 per cent of carers aged between sixteen and thirty-five commenced caring before their sixteenth birthday – a third of whom were caring for a parent: 'This means that of the 1.25 million carers aged 35 and under in 1985, some 212,000 had been providing care since before the age of 16 and, of those, around 68,000 for a parent' (Parker, 1994, p. 9). Analysing OPCS survey data for 1994 Walker (1996) estimates that 32,000 young people aged between eight and eighteen meet the SSI (1995a) definition of 'young carer', although the margin of error imposed by the sampling method-ology means that the actual number of such young people is likely to be between 19,000 and 51,000.

Characteristics of young carers: gender, age and ethnicity

Studies of young carers reflect similar gender patterns to those of the adult population. In the national study of young carers project data, Dearden and Becker (1995) show that 61 per cent and 39 per cent of young carers are female and male respectively; the gender distribution among adult carers being 63 per cent female and 37 per cent male (OPCS, 1992). Given assumptions about gender-appropriate roles, and the view that it is more appropriate for females than males to assume caring roles, it is likely that more girls than boys are young carers in reality. However, it is also possible that these same assumptions may exert particular pressures on boys (fears of teasing, for example,) not to reveal their role as young carers. The extent of caring by young males may, therefore, be under-reported.

Data from young carer projects indicate that many young carers live in a family headed by a lone parent, usually a mother, and that the care recipient is most likely to be the young carer's mother (e.g. Sandwell Caring for Carers, 1989; Aldridge and Becker, 1993; Blyth *et al.*, 1995; Dearden and Becker, 1995; London Borough of Enfield, 1995; Mahon and Higgins, 1995). Dearden and Becker (1995) note that a mother is significantly more likely to be the care recipient in a lone-parent household than in a two-parent household.

This reflects the fact that younger disabled women are considerably more likely to be divorced or separated than both non-disabled women and disabled men (Martin and White, 1988; Lonsdale, 1990). In two-parent families where the father is a care recipient the mother is more likely to provide all or the bulk of care, even if she is also employed outside the home. Where the care recipient is the mother, fathers remaining in the home are less likely to assume a caring role, so children may be more often pulled into providing substitute domestic care especially if the father continues his paid work. It is also more likely that girls rather than boys will undertake caring. Thus, the gender of both the disabled parent and the child are important in the experience of subsequent caring. The absence of a second adult in the household has clear implications for caring for any remaining children.

While a direct causal relationship between disability and marital status has yet to be proven, Mahon and Higgins (1995) observe that there is evidence that for at least some women the onset of their disability or illness triggered the departure of their partner. Quite apart from any other impact which disability in the family has for its members (see below) households headed by a disabled parent are likely to be less well off financially than those where the parent is not disabled. The partners of disabled women may have to give up paid work and families become doubly disabled as both home-making and breadwinning capacities are reduced (Blaxter, 1976; Morris, 1989; Parker, 1993). In addition family income is likely to be more severely affected if the mother is disabled since a disabled woman is less likely than a disabled man to be entitled to contributory and occupational benefits, industrial disablement benefits or compensation payments (Parker, 1993).

To some extent the age profile of young carers will be dependent on the source(s) of their identification, e.g. the clientele of health visitors and schools will be considerably different. However, data from a range of studies provide some general similarities. While there is evidence of some children under the age of five years undertaking caring tasks, the majority are older. Mahon and Higgins (1995) note that most young carers known to the projects they evaluated were aged between eleven and eighteen; Dearden and Becker (1995) state that half of young carers were aged between eleven and fifteen. Blyth *et al.* (1995) report a clustering at ages eleven and twelve, slightly lower than that reported by the London Borough of Enfield (1995) which found that most young carers were aged between twelve and thirteen. (The reported mean age of young carers ranges between ten years and 13.8 years. Where figures are calculated separately for boys and girls, the mean age of male carers appears slightly lower than that for females (11.3 years and 12.4 years (Blyth *et al.*, 1995); and 13.5 years and 13.8 years (Mahon and Higgins, 1995)). Nationally, Dearden and Becker (1995) calculate the mean age of both male and female young carers to be twelve years.

From the national data Dearden and Becker (1995) observe that over 90 per cent of identified young carers are white and conclude that carers projects generally fail to meet the needs of minority ethnic communities.

The difficulties of 'accessing' minority ethnic communities – and hence the under-calculation of young carers from minority ethnic groups – has been noted by several observers (McCalman, 1990; Aldridge and Becker, 1993). However, higher numbers of minority ethnic young carers have been identified where an explicit attempt has been made to access minority ethnic communities. For example, in the Kirklees study, where one of the project staff was an Asian woman, non-white young people comprised 33 per cent (1995) and 41 per cent (1996) of the total number of identified carers (Blyth *et al.*, 1995, 1996). Dearden and Becker (1995) note that young carers from minority ethnic households are more likely to provide intimate care – 35 per cent – compared to 23 per cent of white households. They are also significantly more likely (20 per cent compared to 3 per cent) to be caring for someone other than a parent or a sibling. This may be due to lack of service provision, itself resulting from assumptions that black communities will care for relatives without external support or intervention.

Illness/disability of the care recipient

Care recipients experience a range of physical and mental health problems. As might be expected the largest single group (up to 60 per cent) experience physical ill health or disability. Both Dearden and Becker (1995) and Mahon and Higgins (1995) comment on the relatively high incidence of multiple sclerosis within this category, an illness which is most commonly diagnosed between the ages of 25 and 35, and where any children in the family are likely to be young (Segal and Simkins, 1993). Sensory impairment and learning difficulties each account for a smaller proportion – approximately 6 to 7 per cent each. Of particular note in the studies reported is the high proportion of young carers living with and caring for a relative with mental health problems or those related to alcohol or drug use. Mahon and Higgins (1995) report that nearly half of all young carers were in this position, while slightly lower, but nevertheless still significant, proportions of 34 per cent and 29 per cent were reported by Dearden and Becker (1995) and Blyth *et al.* (1995) respectively.

Mahon and Higgins comment that the sense of emotional labour and burden was especially evident for young carers where there was a mental health problem, including the risks of stigma, teasing and bullying within the neighbourhood and at school.

Tasks performed by young carers

Although, as has been indicated earlier, concern has begun to shift away from an examination of the tasks carried out by young carers to a greater focus on the impact of caring, it is important to establish what young carers do.

First of all are a range of tasks that a parent would normally be expected to perform, such as cooking, cleaning, washing and shopping. These are tasks that all children and young people would generally be expected to undertake to some extent depending on age and ability. What makes undertaking these tasks different for some young carers is their lack of choice (since if they didn't do them no one else could or would) and the extent of their responsibility. In the Kirklees study, for example, some young carers had sole responsibility for the family's weekly shopping, which included not only doing the shopping but budgeting for it and deciding what to buy (Blyth *et al.*, 1995). Dearden and Becker (1995) observe that young carers are more likely to undertake such domestic tasks if the mother is disabled in two-parent households and in households where there is only one parent.

Other 'domestic' tasks undertaken by young carers which other young people are unlikely to be required to do as a matter of routine may include household budgeting, paying bills and collecting benefits, dealing with correspondence, collecting prescriptions and medication.

Where there are other siblings, child-care activities may also fall to another child or young person in the family, particularly in lone-parent households. Common tasks include getting children up, washed and dressed, preparing breakfast and taking them to school, as well as collecting them from school at the end of the afternoon. In the Kirklees study one girl of primary school age recounted her daily routine: 'Just before I go to school I find their school uniform. Sometimes we have to go in normal clothes because we don't know where the shirts are and things like that, so like on the night before we go to school normally now I go and find the clothes for (younger sister and brother) . . . and I help them get dressed . . . I take them to school and pick them up. . . . We have playtime after tea. . . . I sometimes – if it's time – give them a bath and a drink and I put them to bed' (Blyth *et al.*, 1995, p. 23).

Care of a sibling who is disabled may also be undertaken by another child or young person in the family.

Care for the disabled or ill family member may be provided at different levels. First, there is general practical help such as helping with lifting, mobility, accompanying to doctor's or hospital appointments, on shopping or (rarely) leisure trips, cooking, providing drinks and meals, and 'keeping an eye on' the care recipient. The young carer may also have assumed responsibility for deciding when it is necessary to seek medical or other help. Children and young people in black and minority ethnic communities are frequently expected to act as interpreters and liaise with professionals even in the most personal matters regarding the care of a parent (King's Fund Centre, undated).

Second, there are tasks of a more personal and intimate nature, such as brushing and combing hair, washing, dressing, helping in and out of bed, helping with exercises, helping to get to the toilet or to get in and out of a bath or shower, changing medical dressings and administering medication and injections. Mahon and Higgins (1995) note that young carers providing personal care were also more likely to be the main carers and were more likely to be involved in practical caring tasks.

The third category of direct help to the care recipient is emotional support. This may range from keeping them company to listening to their problems and 'trying to cheer them up'. There is evidence that, while such caring is more amorphous than the performance of practical tasks, it may be particularly demanding to young carers, especially where the care recipient has a mental health problem (Mahon and Higgins, 1995). One young carer in Kirklees commented: '(it) has made me really run down and it has affected my school and college work' (Blyth *et al.*, 1995, p. 24).

Dearden and Becker (1995) observe that there is a clear correlation between the nature of the care recipient's illness or disability and the type of care provided. For example, intimate care is most likely to be provided where the care recipient has a physical illness or disability and least likely to be provided where they have a mental health problem, while emotional support is more likely to be provided where the care recipient has a mental health problem and least likely where they have a learning difficulty.

The impact of caring on young carers' lives

A dominant image of caring by young people is one of 'courage', 'self-sacrifice' and 'lost childhood'. Aldridge and Becker (1993) claim that very few young carers have a choice about caring or enjoy their caring roles. Young carers themselves, while acknowledging problems associated with the 'daily physical and financial struggle of caring ... did not want their lives portrayed as nothing but drudgery and despair' (*Community Care* and Carers National Association, 1995, p. 15). Some young carers have normalised their caring role: 'I was a bit worried but I thought "it's part of life. These things happen"' (male carer cited in Blyth *et al.*, 1995, p. 26). Neither are the effects of caring invariably negative ones for the carer. Caring may encourage maturity, self-esteem, responsibility and independence (Bowis, 1995) and young carers often derive positive feedback from their caring relationship (Aldridge and Becker, 1993). While research evidence does suggest that caring may pose particular problems for young carers or restrict their lives or development in some way, similar problems, resulting from poverty or family dynamics, could be experienced by other children not formally identified as young carers.

As we have already noted one of the reasons advanced for the inadequacy of knowledge about young carers is the belief that fear of the consequences of discovery by statutory agencies may inhibit young carers and care recipients from advertising the existence of their particular circumstances (Aldridge and Becker, 1993, 1994; *Community Care* and Carers National Association, 1995). While such fears do exist, their prevalence should not be exaggerated (Blyth *et al.*, 1995; Mahon and Higgins, 1995).

As we have already indicated, illness and disability may impact on roles and responsibilities within the family, although we would not wish to promote assumptions that caring by children and young people will necessarily have an adverse impact on parenting. Disabled rights activists have argued that parenting involves more than the performance of physical tasks conventionally carried out by parents and that the inability to carry these out does not diminish a disabled parent's ability to love and care for their child, let alone constitute 'role reversal' between parent and child (Keith and Morris, 1995; Mahon and Higgins, 1995; Olsen, 1996). In order to avoid these difficulties the Social Services Inspectorate (1996) suggests that it is useful to distinguish between support for 'parenting' (concern for the child's welfare) and support for 'parental activity' (the tasks parents do as parents). The financial disadvantage experienced by many families where a parent has a disability may also have a profound effect on all family members (*Community Care* and Carers National Association, 1995).

Stigma, or fear of it, appears to be a frequent experience of young carers (Blyth *et al.*, 1995; Mahon and Higgins, 1995; SSI, 1996) as illustrated by Nicola, a fifteen-year-old young carer participating in a conference organised by *Community Care* magazine and the Carers National Association: 'You can't tell your friends or people at school because they will pick on you. You are scared that if people find out you look after someone, there will be a lot of whispering because they don't understand' (*Community Care* and Carers National Association, 1995, p. 14). Mahon and Higgins (1995) also note that teasing or bullying at school, directly related to the young person's caring role or to an ill or disabled family member, may result in absence from school.

Leisure activities, too, may be constrained by the tasks which young carers undertake. In the Kirklees study, for example, several young carers felt that they could not play outdoors too far from home in case they were needed, so they had to remain within shouting distance at least. Others had managed to organise one or two evenings a week of 'respite' when they could go out knowing that someone else was keeping an eye on things at home. One young carer described the balance which she had to strike between her own leisure interests and those of younger siblings who needed transporting or escorting to various activities (Blyth *et al.*, 1995).

As already noted, for some young carers the illness or disability of a parent or other family member or involvement in caring activities may have a profound effect on their education. This may be associated with punctuality and attendance, poor concentration because of stress or tiredness and difficulty in completing classwork and homework. Becker and Aldridge (1995) calculate that a quarter of school-age young carers are missing school. Absence from school as a result of caring may be intermittent, depending on particular circumstances from day to day. Otherwise absence may be occasional but regular (e.g. in order to accompany a care recipient for hospital appointments) or complete (e.g. during a crisis or period of acute illness).

Young carers may find it difficult to concentrate on classwork or homework because of the need to juggle demands of school with those of home and consequent tiredness as a result of work which had to be done at home or because of worry about a sick or disabled parent: 'Sometimes I feel like falling asleep in class but I know I've got to get on with my studies' (young carer cited in Blyth *et al.*, 1995, p. 27); 'I was really forgetful because I was thinking about what was happening with my mum and things like that. Because I didn't know what was happening. And then at the time of her operation I was just spaced out. I didn't think about anything else' (young carer cited in Blyth *et al.*, 1995, p. 26).

Just as some young carers express concern about the potential or actual responses of peers and friends, so too are there concerns about the way teachers may recognise and respond to young carers. Young carers participating in the national conference organised by *Community Care* magazine and the Carers National Association considered it was not helpful for teachers to identify them publicly, however genuine the motivation and intention (*Community Care* and Carers National Association, 1995).

A final aspect of the educational experience of young carers is the recognition of school as a 'haven', a place where they can be treated as children and where they can enjoy a respite from the demands of domestic and caring responsibilities (Bilsborrow, 1992; Dearden and Becker, 1995). What is implicit in raising the negative aspects of caring is the amount of time young people spend on caring activities. Out of 14 young carers aged between twelve and seventeen interviewed by the Office for National Statistics (Walker, 1996) 9 were spending more than 20 hours each week (and averaging 3 hours each day) and 2 young people were spending 32 hours a week on caring. Although caring in the home is not covered by children's employment legislation (see chapter 10) it is of note that this imposes limits of 2 hours' work each school day for children of compulsory school age. Over a week no child under the age of 15 years should be employed for more than fifteen hours, and no child between fifteen years and compulsory school-leaving age should be employed for more than 30 hours.

Legislation and policy

Whether or not individual children or young people meet the narrower SSI definition of 'young carer' should be largely irrelevant. The best interests of children should be a 'primary consideration in all actions concerning children whether undertaken by public or private social welfare institutions' (United Nations Convention on the Rights of the Child, 1989) and several Articles of the Convention safeguard in principle the rights of young carers (Children's Rights Development Unit, 1994; Farrington of Ribbleton, 1995).

Child care, community care and carers legislation in Britain should already provide a sufficiently broad legislative framework to facilitate service provision for young carers, although it is for local authorities themselves to decide how to ensure integrated service provision, through coordinated Community Care Plans and Children's Services Plans (SSI, 1995a, 1996). The NHS and Community Care Act 1990 places on local authorities responsibilities to ensure the provision of effective services for disabled people in order to maintain them in their own homes. Under the Act service users have a right to advocacy and representation, separate assessment of the needs of the carer and the care recipient may be provided and carers may request an assessment to be made.

Carers' rights to an assessment have further statutory backing through the Carers (Recognition and Services) Act 1995. Under the provisions of this Act a carer is defined as an individual providing a 'substantial amount of care on a regular basis' for someone who is 'blind, deaf or dumb (or who suffers from mental disorder of any description) and other persons (aged eighteen or over) who are substantially and permanently handicapped by illness, injury, or congenital deformity or such other disabilities as may be prescribed by the Minister' (National Assistance Act 1948, Section 29).

Under the Act, local authority social services departments have a duty to assess the ability of a carer to provide and continue to provide care when deciding what services should be provided to the care recipient. The Act does not define carers in terms of either their age or their relationship to the person they care for and the Department of Health has produced specific guidance on the application of the Act to young carers for those undertaking assessment and providing services (DOH, 1995a, b). Principal characteristics of the recommended approach are: respect for the integrity of the family; focus on the family as a whole; acknowledgement of the way the family has coped with the illness or disability of a family member; seeing young carers as 'children first'; avoidance of undermining parenting capacity; and recognition that parents' and children's views and interests may not be the same.

Under the Act, young carers may request an assessment in their own right. If an assessment reveals that the young carer is being subjected to considerable burdens the local authority has a duty to increase the level of service provision to the care recipient, although there are several important caveats. First, how the term 'substantial' should be applied to young, as opposed to adult, carers in order to avoid young carers being required to assume age-inappropriate responsibilities. Second, that an explicit focus on providing personal care for the ill or disabled person should not become excessively task-oriented and lead to other caring activities, especially less tangible aspects such as the provision of emotional support, undertaking general (but excessive) household duties and childcare tasks, and which appear integral to the lives of many young carers, being overlooked. Third, since the triggers for carer assessment are assessment or re-assessment of the care recipient, how the needs of existing young carers can be addressed, particularly if the care recipient refuses an assessment.

Alternatively the extent and impact of their caring responsibilities may result in young carers being regarded as children 'in need' and eligible for services under the provisions of the Children Act 1989, particularly where they are not providing care on a 'regular or substantial basis' or where they are otherwise affected by the illness or disability of a family member.

The five major principles of the Children Act as elucidated in subsequent guidance – focus on the welfare of the child; partnership with parents; the importance of families; the importance of the views of children and their parents, and the corporate responsibility of local authority – can be related to young carers.

Under the Children Act 1989 every local authority has a duty (a) to safeguard and promote the welfare of children within their area who are 'in need' and (b) so far as is consistent with that duty, to promote the upbringing of such children by their families, by providing a range and level of services appropriate to those children's needs (S. 17[1]). Under Section 17 (10) a child is considered to be 'in need' if:

- they are unlikely to achieve or maintain or to have opportunity of achieving or maintaining a reasonable standard of health or development without the provision for them of services by a local authority, or
- their health or development is likely to be significantly impaired, or further impaired, without the provision for them of such services.

(The third group of children 'in need' under the Act – disabled children – are considered in more detail in chapter 8.)

It is for local authorities to decide whether groups of children and young people (such as young carers) or individual children and young people meet the definition of a child 'in need'.

Such assessment of need should be undertaken in an open way and should involve those caring for the child and other significant persons and, where possible, should enable children and young people to participate in the decision-making process about their future well-being (DOH, 1989, 2:2.7; 2.28).

Where children are recognised as being 'in need' they are entitled to services that should be provided under Schedule 2, paragraph 8 of the Children Act. These are identified as:

- advice, guidance and counselling;
- occupational, social, cultural and recreational activities;
- home help (including laundry facilities);
- facilities or assistance with travelling to and from any services provided under the Act or any similar service, and
- assistance to enable the child and the family to have a holiday.

Local authorities are empowered to 'put together a package of services for a family which could include home help, day-care provision for a family member other than the child in need, or a short-term, temporary placement for the child', where the services are provided to promote the child's welfare (DOH, 1989, 2:2.6).

Other provisions of the Children Act which may have a bearing on official responses to young carers are those relating to child protection. Bentovim (1991) refers to children who are 'inducted into parental caretaking roles' and children who are deprived of opportunities to develop relationships with peers or to play and whose personal development is restricted as 'emotionally abused'. Children undertaking physical caring tasks, such as lifting, may be put at risk of physical injury (impairment of physical development). Young people who live with parents who misuse drugs and alcohol, who have mental health problems or learning difficulties may well fall within the remit of the child protection system. Some observers have noted that a more punitive or reactionary form of intervention may be taken in such families (Weir, 1994; Alexander, 1995; Wallace, 1995; Waddell, 1996). Indeed, given that the focus of social services' child-care provision is child protection rather than children 'in need', it is unlikely that young carers will receive much priority for assistance as children 'in need', and social work intervention via the child protection route may result in services taking over the care of the child rather than helping the parent manage childcare (SSI 1995b, p. 12).

Indeed, a major conclusion from research studies, consultation events and accounts of individual experiences, is that, rather than being afforded special consideration, young carers are *less* likely than their adult counterparts to receive either appropriate community support or community care services. Sylvia Heal, Young Carers Project Officer at Carers National Association, stated: 'Probably the most significant problems researchers identified was the feeling of young carers that nobody listened to what they had to say' (SSI, 1995b, p. 15).

Becker (1993), reporting on the Nottingham study, comments that not only were young carers less likely to receive informal support and help from neighbours and family but, if anything, the response of professionals was even worse. In particular, domiciliary services were withdrawn when young carers were considered old enough to cope. Becker's censure of the education welfare service's punitive treatment of young carers who were not attending school is echoed by David Hinchliffe MP, recalling his own days as a social worker in Leeds: 'I can recall cases of non-school attendance that brought the circumstances of a child or young person to the attention of local authorities. Those young people were then seen as the problem, and not part of a much wider issue. . . . I am shamed to admit that I can recall several children being taken before juvenile courts who were found to be young carers. They were not at school because they were carrying out difficult caring tasks. It is not right that they should be seen as the problem' (Hinchliffe, 1995). (It should not escape the reader's attention that Hinchliffe is referring to practices occurring when the Leeds adjournment system was flourishing.)

Reinforcing the Audit Commission's (1994) view that community health, education and social services are generally poorly coordinated and the SSI (1996) description of services provided to young carers and their families as 'unco-ordinated' and 'unpredictable', one young carer in Kirklees who, asked if he knew of any services which might provide help, replied: 'the only organisation I've heard of is "help yourself" – which is me' (Blyth *et al.*, 1995, p. 25).

Good practice

The achievement of the young carers movement has been to push young carers further up the political agenda. Many areas now have established local young carers' services, often provided on an inter-agency basis, which have served to establish the identity of young carers and have begun to provide child-centred services which are responsive to their needs. Furthermore, it is important to recognise that without such initiatives it is unlikely that the young people or their families would have received any assistance at all. One of the consistent themes from the young carers research is that the young people were already known to at least one person in an official position or voluntary organisation and still received inadequate help. However, most if not all young carers' projects are subject to the vagaries of short-term funding and the insecurity regarding longer term planning and service delivery which this entails. In addition the SSI (1996) notes the variable quality of local authority young carers policy statements and the potential problems of projects being seen as 'dumping grounds', and subject to unrealistic expectations, including the assumption of local authorities' care management and coordination responsibilities.

Disability rights activists have been critical of the development of the 'young carers' movement', arguing that the focus on young carers has reinforced the image of disabled people – especially mothers – as dependent and incapable of exercising autonomy and has conveniently shifted attention away from the provision of adequate support for the disabled (Keith and Morris, 1995; Olsen, 1996). They argue that the category of 'young carer' is an artificial creation which reinforces pressures on families and informal networks to enable disabled people to live in the community with minimal formal support, and that the young carers 'mission' effectively ignores the socio-economic disadvantage and lack of appropriate support which propel children and young people into becoming carers. If these issues were faced squarely the need for children and young people to provide care and for them to carry out inappropriate tasks – some of which may place them at physical risk – would be prevented. Furthermore, official hand-wringing over what are reasonable or acceptable levels of 'responsibility' for children is based on a total misconception about the nature of parenting and the ability of disabled parents to exercise parental responsibility. If services were made available which empowered disabled parents to carry out their parental responsibilities there would be less risk of undermining the disabled parent's role as a parent and of 'blaming' disabled parents for having to rely on their children for support. One crucial area which disability rights activists appear to gloss over is the possibility of a conflict of interest between a disabled parent and a potential or actual young carer, which is not simply resolved by the availability of support from outside the family. For example, offers of assistance with potentially embarrassing intimate personal tasks may be rejected in favour of help from a family carer regardless of whether the carer wishes to provide such a help. Young carers in this position may, in practice, have little choice about what help they are expected to provide.

The resource implications of the disability rights perspective are, therefore, at odds with the message from young carers research, that appropriate support would make few demands on resources because young carers' needs are relatively limited – they want the opportunity to be listened to, to talk to someone, to 'let off steam', and to share their worries and fears, rather than expensive support services. 'Experience shows that extending choice and power for families does not necessarily stretch budgets – the needs expressed are often about organisational arrangements and have minimal financial demands' (SSI, 1995b, p.18).

Given these tensions, what should be the most appropriate way forward? In the plethora of advice and guidance, several key themes emerge which policy-makers and professionals across agency boundaries need to take on board. There is an evident need for a coordinated multi-disciplinary approach to service provision and practice which transcends agency boundaries and, within local authorities, traditionally separate services for children and adults. The Social Services Inspectorate is encouraging such developments 'through clearly identified links' between Children's Services and Community Care Plans and in some areas joint commissioning and joint finance have been used to promote these. Services should be seen as non-stigmatising and non-threatening to the disabled person, young carer and other family members. Priority for services must be to ensure that disabled parents are supported in exercising their parental responsibilities. Schools, for example, could ensure that their facilities are accessible for disabled parents. Any caring tasks undertaken by children and young people should be ones over which they exercise choice and control. Young people should not have to perform tasks they do not wish to undertake and which may put them at risk. As we have already noted, it is important to recognise that the needs and wishes of a disabled parent and those of an actual or potential young carer may not always be identical. One way in which pressures can be lifted from potential young carers is a policy decision, taken by at least some local authorities, that anyone being cared for by a person under the age of eighteen is to be considered to have no carer and is therefore eligible to receive the same care as those with no informal carer (SSI, 1996).

All professionals and workers in voluntary organisations working with children or with sick or disabled adults or children should be aware of the possibility that illness or disability in a family may exert a physical or emotional impact on children in the family. It should not be assumed that statutory or voluntary agencies with whom the family may be in contact will necessarily be 'young carer aware'. Teachers and education welfare officers are in particularly 'good' positions to identify young carers and ensure that they are aware of appropriate services and receive necessary support (NASWE, 1994; Mahon and Higgins, 1995; Farrington of Ribbleton, 1995; SSI, 1996).

CHAPTER 7

School attendance

Introduction

Despite the fact that most young people of school age in this country both attend school regularly and recognise the personal benefits to themselves of a sound education (e.g. O'Keeffe, 1994; Hughes and Lloyd, 1996), politicians and the media appear caught up in a moral panic about levels of non-attendance, its presumed link with delinquency, and young people's rejection of education (e.g. DFE, 1992a; Scott-Clark and Burke, 1996; Scott-Clark and Syal, 1996). While it is true that the immediate and longer-term consequences of missing extensive periods of schooling may be profound, exaggerating the scale and impact of the problem may also be counter-productive. On a national scale it is impossible to compare current attendance or absence levels with those of the past; the standards of attendance registration in British schools are such that there are 'no nationally usable statistics' (DES, 1989b) and no evidence of any significant deterioration in attendance levels (Reid, 1985). Human error and post-registration truancy (O'Keeffe, 1994) apart, we noted in chapter 1 the risk of attendance registers being 'rigged' to improve the pay of teachers and head teachers. The school's position in performance tables and its 'image' have replaced teachers' pay as incentives to present published attendance data in the most favourable light (i.e. redesignating ostensibly 'unauthorised' absence as 'authorised' absence). And even if we were confident of the accuracy of attendance data, overall absence levels reveal little useful information. A given absence rate could, for example, be indicative of a large number of pupils missing small amounts of school or a very small number of pupils permanently – or almost permanently – absent. However, for the pupils in the latter group, the consequences of truancy are grave.

Prevalence and patterns

Official records, therefore, are not necessarily useful in measuring the prevalence of truancy. Estimates range widely, the *Guardian* (1990), for example, reporting 'more than half a million children' absent at least once a week without 'acceptable reason' (cited in Gleeson, 1992), while in 1995 the public sector union Unison was claiming that over 800,000 children a year 'played truant' (cited in Montgomery, 1996). The plethora of definitions and categorisations of absence from school used by different researchers and writers makes detailed comparison between research studies virtually impossible. Even dedicated truancy studies (e.g. O'Keeffe, 1994) using self-reporting measures, may well underestimate true levels since they are least likely to identify the young people most likely to be absent from school.

For example, Stoll and O'Keeffe (1989), who interviewed pupils at school, found two thirds of pupils admitting to truanting at some time during their secondary schooling, although only about 30 per cent of pupils admitted to so doing in O'Keeffe's later study (O'Keeffe, 1994). 'Post-registration' truancy, i.e. absence from lessons after pupils have registered in school appears to be more prevalent than 'blanket' truancy, although many truants are engaged in both (Stoll and O'Keeffe, 1989; O'Keeffe, 1994). A small minority of pupils appear to be 'frequent truants', O'Keeffe identifying 2.5 per cent (Year 10) and 4.5 per cent (Year 11) pupils who admitted to truanting at least once a week, while Gray and Jesson (1990) found that 6 per cent of Year 11 pupils were absent for days or weeks at a time, and Farrington (1996) notes that by the ages of twelve to fourteen, 18 per cent of his (all male) sample were identified by teachers as either 'frequent truants' (although 'frequency' is not defined) or had poor attendance attributed to truancy, while at age fourteen a similar percentage admitted 'frequent truancy'.

Truancy rates typically increase during the last two years of compulsory schooling, peaking in Year 11 in an English study (O'Keeffe, 1994) and S4 in a Scottish study (SCRE, 1992). O'Keeffe (1994) found that slightly more boys than girls admitted to truanting: 24.6 per cent of Year 10 boys; 25.5 per cent of Year 10 girls; 37.7 per cent of Year 11 boys; 30.5 per cent of Year 11 girls. However, he reports that truancy levels at single-sex boys' schools tend to be higher than at mixed schools, with single-sex girls' schools having consistently lower levels of truancy than either mixed or single-sex boys' schools. Carlen *et al.* (1992) note that girls are more likely than boys to be involved in condoned absence.

The causes of truancy

The results of several decades of research indicate that, although evidence of direct causal relationships is elusive, there is a correlation between truancy and individual, peer group, family, neighbourhood and school factors.

Historically, the search for the causes of truancy has focused on individual and family factors (e.g. O'Keeffe, 1994; Casey and Smith, 1995; Farrington, 1996; Graham and Bowling, 1995). O'Keeffe (1994) and Graham and Bowling (1995) identify a strong relationship between truancy and parental supervision and family attachment. Graham and Bowling also note that the likelihood of truanting is increased by two to three times in families characterised by 'weak' parental supervision and 'low' family attachment, while O'Keeffe identifies the connection between adverse socio-economic factors and high levels of absence.

By the early 1980s the focus of attention had shifted substantially to the impact of the education system and schools as research on school effectiveness demonstrated the strong relationship between disruptive behaviour and persistent non-attendance and the organisation and ethos of particular schools, irrespective of the individual characteristics of their pupils and their pupils' families. Positively, this research suggests that well supported schools can help to combat the impact of adverse family and social factors (e.g. Rutter *et al.*, 1979; Mortimore *et al.*, 1988a; Graham, 1992; Reynolds and Cuttance, 1992). Specific in-school factors which are associated with non-attendance include bullying (Learmonth, 1995) and curricular difficulties (O'Keeffe, 1994). On occasions reluctance to attend school may be to avoid being abused by a teacher (e.g. Cornwall County Council, 1987). Learmonth, (1995) indicates that the develop- ment of in-school anti-bullying schemes may contribute to improved school attendance by making schools more congenial environments for children. O'Keeffe's finding that, according to pupils' own accounts, the most important source of truancy is the school curriculum itself is reinforced by Learmonth (1995). OFSTED (1995a) found a high correlation between rates of attendance and pupil performance in public examinations, high rates of attendance accompanying success in public examinations and low levels of attendance accompanying unsatisfactory or poor examination results. These findings reinforce contentions (e.g. Grenville, 1988; Holmes, 1989) that absenteeism may on occasions at least represent a rational consumer response to dissatisfaction with the service on offer.

O'Keeffe's study supports this suggestion, as the most common reason given by truants for truanting was the wish to avoid particular lessons. Specific components of dissatisfaction with lessons included lack of enjoyment found in lessons, irrelevance of lessons or excessive difficulty and the unlikeable personalities of some teachers. This study also revealed that different subjects were affected by different levels of truancy. Maths – the least favourite subject – was avoided by 22 per cent of truants, while only 3 per cent admitting to missing Technology. Rejection of specific lessons, though, is accompanied by recognition by most young people of school age, including truants, of the intrinsic value of education (O'Keeffe, 1994; Hughes and Lloyd, 1996).

Outcomes of truancy

There is a long research tradition in this country which has observed an association between truancy and juvenile crime. However, despite political and ideological rhetoric, evidence of a causative relationship between truancy and delinquency remains elusive, and some researchers have wondered whether the relationship has more to do with truancy and delinquency themselves having common causes.

Some caution should be exercised in interpreting some of the research data. For example, the research conducted by Graham and Bowling (1995) and Farrington (1996), while providing useful insights, is primarily concerned with young people's offending behaviour rather than truancy. Although direct comparisons between these two studies are difficult to make because they use different criteria to define 'truancy', are based on young people of different ages, and the subjects of Farrington's study are exclusively male, their findings identify similar patterns. They reveal significant overlaps between truancy and juvenile delinquency. In Farrington's study 48 per cent of secondary school truants had criminal convictions, compared with 14 per cent of non-truants, while Graham and Bowling report that 37 per cent of their male respondents and 28 per cent of female respondents admitted to absenting themselves from school without authorisation for at least one day. Both male and female truants were three times more likely than non-truants to offend. Those who persistently truanted were even more likely to admit offending (78 per cent of males and 53 per cent of females who truanted once a week committed offences). Graham and Bowling also note that the onset of truancy and delinquency occur around the same time (the average age at which both males and females started offending was 13.5, while the average age for the onset of truancy was 13.5 for females and 14 for males). However, they acknowledge that their data do not prove a causal relationship between truancy and offending. In Farrington's study there was almost complete matching between truancy and delinquency of significantly related social and personal variables, leading to the conclusion that 'truancy and delinquency are two behavioural symptoms of an anti-social personality' (Farrington, 1996, p. 115). Other research suggests a link between non-attendance and sexual offending. Kahn and Chambers (1991) found that half their sample of sex offenders had histories of disruptive behaviour, one third had a history of truancy and two thirds had learning difficulties, while O'Callaghan and Print (1994) found a long history of truancy to be a contra-indication for community-based treatment of adolescent sex offenders.

Noting the gender patterns of truancy and crime, O'Keeffe observes: 'Juvenile delinquency is undoubtedly predominantly male in character. But if truancy is not especially male-dominated, while juvenile crime is, the notion of a causal nexus between truancy and delinquency needs to be treated rather cautiously' (O'Keeffe, 1994, p. 89). Lewis (1995) notes that while persistent young offenders are responsible for a high volume of crime, it would be a mistake to assume that 'all children in shopping centres are involved in criminal activities' (Lewis, 1995, p. 21). He also recognises that official crime data show that only a minority of truants are convicted of crimes, citing a Home Office survey of shopkeepers in two Midlands shopping complexes which highlighted shopkeepers' perceptions of youths being mainly involved in incidents of 'gathering' and 'loitering'. Most reported thefts were committed by adults, not juveniles. Lewis's own survey, which sought to find out where truants went and what they did when truanting, revealed that the majority of truants 'do nothing in particular' (Lewis, 1995, p. 24). This research did reveal the potential vulnerability of truants, while truanting, to threats, theft, and to physical and sexual abuse (see later on 'Truancy Watch').

Casey and Smith (1995), reporting on the England and Wales Youth Cohort Study, conclude that, for young people between the ages of sixteen and nineteen there is a strong correlation between truancy and poor outcomes in education, training and the labour market. Two major longitudinal studies, the National Child Development Study (Hibbett *et al.*, 1990; Hibbett and Fogelman, 1990) and the Cambridge Study in Delinquent Development (Farrington and West, 1990; Farrington, 1996) provide further evidence of the longer-term negative effects of truancy into early adulthood.

Analysis of NCDS data, when the cohort were aged twenty-three, by Hibbett *et al.* (1990) and Hibbett and Fogelman (1990) indicates that, after controlling for the effects of social background, educational ability, poor attendance due to other factors, and end-of-school qualifications, former truants differed from their non-truanting peers in a number of key occupational and social areas. They were more likely to have lower-status occupations, less stable career patterns and higher levels of unemployment. They were also more likely to have been younger at the time of the birth of their first child, have had more children, have experienced marital breakdown, and more likely to be heavy smokers and to suffer depression. The authors do not consider that these findings support the idea that truants simply outgrow school and are ready for the world of work or that the difficulties they experience reflect a quicker rate of progress through the major events and transitions of early adulthood. Rather they point to the continuing effect of psychological problems previously evident during truants' adolescence.

The Cambridge Study in Delinquent Development is a prospective longitudinal study of the development of offending and anti-social behaviour in 411 London males who were first contacted in 1961–2 when they were aged eight or nine. Farrington (1996) notes that at the ages of eighteen and again at thirty-two those who had truanted while at school characteristically engaged in a range of anti-social behaviours. The findings regarding employment histories are similar to those of the National Child Development Study, with truants tending to have low status (unskilled manual) jobs and an unstable job record. There is a significant overlap between truancy and juvenile delinquency; 48 per cent of secondary school truants were convicted, compared with 14 per cent of non-truants. Every variable significantly related to delinquency was also significantly related to truancy and every variable, except for a low social class family at age eight to ten, that was significantly related to truancy was also significantly related to delinquency. Longer-term correlations with poor educational experiences are also evidenced in the National Prison Survey (1991) showing that 43 per cent of prisoners had left school before the age of sixteen, including 1 per cent who claimed they had never attended school (Walmsley *et al*., 1992), leading to suggestions that positive crime-reduction measures schools can take are to tackle under-achievement and reduce absence from school resulting from both truancy and exclusion and (see also chapter 9) (Audit Commission, 1996b; NACRO, 1997).

School attendance, the law and policy

Every child in Britain aged between five (four in Northern Ireland) and sixteen is required to receive 'efficient, full-time education suitable to (their) age, ability, aptitude and to any special educational needs (they) may have'. Most children will receive their education through attendance at a state school, although a few are educated at independent schools. In addition the law allows for children to be educated other than by attendance at school so long as their parents can provide evidence of the suitability of the education being provided.

If a child is not registered at a school and the education authority establishes that they are not being properly educated 'otherwise' it may serve a notice requiring the child's parent(s) to register the child at a school of their choosing. If the parents fail to respond to this notice within a given time the child will be registered at a school chosen by the education authority. Parents who subsequently fail to secure the regular attendance of the child at the school at which they are registered are guilty of an offence. The maximum fine upon conviction is £1,000.

The law provides a number of defence grounds: that the child was absent with leave; the child was ill or prevented from attending by any unavoidable cause; the absence was due to religious observance; the school at which the child is a registered pupil is not within walking distance of the child's home and appropriate transport arrangements were not made by the LEA; and the family has a travelling lifestyle (in which case the child must attend for a minimum of two hundred sessions (half days) during the preceding twelve months).

Despite the establishment of a considerable body of case law the category of absence 'with leave' has proved problematic. In order to clarify this the government introduced two new categories of absence, 'authorised' and 'unauthorised' (DFE, 1994f). Absence may only be 'authorised' by the school, not the child's parent(s). If absence is authorised by the school then no offence is committed. Any absence which is not authorised is, by definition, unauthorised. There remains considerable discretion over which absences schools may authorise despite regulations and guidance, although more detailed guidance than that issued by the DFE has been issued to Scottish schools, education authorities and parents (SOED, 1995). In English schools there remains continuing ambiguity about the categorisation of absences and the powers to authorise it (OFSTED, 1995a, b); again undermining the credibility of published absence data. The element of discretion about the categorisation of absence is somewhat controversial, especially when details of unauthorised absences were first required to be included in published performance data in 1993. Some schools which considered they had conscientiously applied government guidance on the categorisation of absence complained that they had been penalised in 'league' table terms in comparison with schools which had adopted a less rigorous approach to absence categorisation (OFSTED, 1995a).

A further twist in this particular 'tale' is that while truancy is categorised as unauthorised absence, exclusion from school is recognised as authorised absence (although in Scotland exclusion is deemed to be unauthorised absence, also highlighting procedural inconsistencies between UK jurisdictions). Therefore, despite an unambiguous message from the DFE that 'exclusion is not an appropriate response to . . . irregular attendance' (DFE, 1994d, p. 12) schools in England and Wales have been able to convert a major source of unauthorised absence to authorised absence by formally excluding truants. Further attempts to 'improve' attendance statistics to which schools have resorted include enforced parental 'withdrawal' of unwelcome pupils, informal (illegal) exclusions, illicit granting of 'study leave' and removing absent pupils from school rolls (OFSTED, 1995a; Stirling, 1996).

There are two legal approaches open to education authorities to enforce school attendance. They may prosecute parents under provisions of the relevant education legislation or they may take action in respect of the child under child-care legislation. Despite some differences between the different jurisdictions broadly similar measures exist throughout the UK. In exceptional circumstances non-attendance alone could satisfy the 'significant harm' test necessary for an application by a local authority for a care order under the provisions of the Children Act 1989. Robertson (1996) suggests that the ruling in *Re* O (1992), that failure to attend school can amount to 'significant harm', opens up the possibility of social services, in consultation with the LEA, making use of other provisions under the Act, for example, a Child Assessment Order or even using non-attendance as the basis for an application for an Emergency Protection Order.

Strategies for non-attenders

Education welfare officers and teachers are well aware that persistent non-attenders are typically those young people in Years 10 and 11, who, over a long period, have been unable to establish regular patterns of attendance within mainstream education, despite sanctions and/or considerable amounts of support from within school and by external agencies. The challenges for professionals concerned with such young people focus on the use of legal and administrative sanctions (and whether or not these are any more than token gestures) and how – if at all – they are to be properly educated.

The former government claimed that the early prosecution of parents may be 'particularly effective', not only in relation to the individual child, but also as a warning to others (DES, 1991b), although failing to provide supporting evidence for this assertion. Statistics produced in 1995 relating to the number of parental prosecutions initiated by English LEAs suggest a less-than-straightforward relationship between LEAs' prosecution and unauthorised absence rates (DFE, 1995b; DFEE, 1995b) albeit providing evidence of increased use of parental prosecution which rose by nearly a third, between 1991–2 (2,803 prosecutions) and 1993–4 (3,688 prosecutions). These statistics show that some LEAs are able to produce low overall rates of unauthorised absence without recourse to legal action at all. Evidence about the impact of parental prosecution in specific local authorities is also sparse, although a report produced by Solihull Metropolitan Borough Council (1992) concluded that parental prosecution was 'ineffective' in its impact on pupil attendance.

It may be that – despite its apparent failure to improve the attendance of those children whose parents are actually prosecuted – parental prosecution may exercise some general deterrent effect or possess symbolic value in setting the boundaries of acceptable behaviour (e.g. Whitney, 1994; OFSTED, 1995a). However, the Solihull study concluded that parental prosecution had no discernible 'knock-on' effect on the attendance pattern of any other children in the family. None of the available data on the outcomes of parental prosecution have been sufficiently rigorously analysed to identify the effectiveness of parental prosecution in particular circumstances, for example, whether 'early' prosecution of the parents of (usually) younger pupils is more effective than the use of court as a sanction of 'last resort'.

The professional association representing magistrates has itself openly expressed concern that prosecutions appear to target poor parents (e.g. Petre, 1994) and scepticism about the efficacy of prosecution: 'The Association is far from convinced that the Adult Court is the proper forum with which to deal with this matter and believes that measures designed to *prevent* truancy would be preferable and probably more effective than any of the disposals realistically available to a criminal court' (Magistrates' Association, 1994 – our emphasis). As an apparent response to the lack of success in parental prosecution influencing school attendance, media reports indicate that some magistrates are applying novel 'solutions' to the problem, although reported instances are rare (e.g. Montgomery, 1996; National Association of Probation Officers, 1996 (personal communication); Scott-Clark and Burke, 1996; White, 1996; Whitehead, 1996). These have included one instance of magistrates placing a mother on probation for failing to send her children to school; and two occasions where magistrates postponed sentencing, placing the parents on bail with a condition that they take the child to school and hand the child over to the teacher. While making probation orders in these instances is itself within the law, the development has been viewed with some concern by the National Association of Probation Officers (personal communication, 1996) and appears to make a parent's failure to secure their child's proper education a more serious offence than that envisaged in education legislation. The use of bail following conviction in such circumstances appears more ambiguous legally, Rodgers (forthcoming) suggesting that deferring sentence for a period of up to six months might have been a more appropriate course of action. The use of both post-sentence bail and sentence deferral would, of course, bear striking similarities to the adjournment procedures implemented by juvenile magistrates in Leeds in the 1970s and would make magistrates the enforcers of school attendance. Whether magistrates wish to assume this role on a far greater scale than the occasional one-off case and whether the initial success of these initiatives will prove more effective in the longer term than existing measures remain to be seen.

Information about the effectiveness of education supervision orders is even less readily available than that for parental prosecution. Circumstances under which a court may impose an education supervision order are circumscribed. Before an LEA applies for an education supervision order 'all reasonable efforts should have been made to resolve a problem of poor school attendance without the use of legal sanctions' (DOH, 1991b, p. 25). The court may only make the order if the child is of compulsory school age and is not being properly educated, although an order cannot be made if the child is already in the care of a local authority. In addition, in keeping with the principles of the Children Act, the court must take account of the welfare of the child (Section 1 [1]), including the factors identified in the welfare checklist requiring the court to take account of the child's ascertainable wishes and feelings, their educational needs, any harm that has been suffered, the capability of the parents in meeting the child's needs and the range of powers available to the court under the Act. The latter include any order which the court may make under Section 8 of the Act, although these are likely to be used infrequently, if at all. Finally, the court needs to be satisfied that making the order will be more beneficial to the child than making no order at all, although, in a High Court ruling (Essex CC *v* B. 1993) it was held that, even if parental cooperation seemed unlikely, the LEA should still consider the possibility of applying for an education supervision order rather than let the situation 'drift'.

Data produced by the government (DFE, 1995b) and NASWE (1996) indicate that few applications for education supervision orders have been made by LEAs (although the number of applications is increasing) compared to the number of parental prosecutions. (It should be noted that while the government data includes all English LEAs, NASWE data is less complete, providing information from 61 English and Welsh LEAs in 1991–2; and 53 and 55 English LEAs in 1992–3 and 1993–4 respectively.)

Between 1991 and 1994 the annual number of education supervision orders granted by courts increased from 81 to 314 (DFE, 1995b). Data from NASWE (1996) show that the success rate of applications made by LEAs for education supervision orders increased from 67.2 per cent in

1991–2 to 80.2 per cent in 1993–4. Over the same period the rate of courts' directions to LEAs to initiate an application for an education supervision order decreased from 8.3 per cent of all prosecutions in 1991–2 to 5.4 per cent in 1993–4, while LEAs' 'compliance rates' increased from 23.9 per cent in 1991–2 to 34.6 per cent in 1993–4, suggesting a gradual convergence of magistrates' and LEAs' positions, possibly as a result of increased familiarity and confidence with the new procedures. To date there have been no studies evaluating the effectiveness of Education Supervision Orders in improving school attendance.

There are a variety of explanations both for the relatively few ESO applications which have been made and for LEAs' preferences for prosecution. The DOH expectation that LEAs should have 'tried everything' before applying for an education supervision order appears responsible for a view within LEAs that there is little to be gained by applying for – and obtaining – an order. Pressures on LEA resources – the financial and administrative costs associated with applying for an order, demonstrating the existence of the necessary criteria for making an order and outlining a detailed action plan – may act as a further disincentive. By comparison, parental prosecution may be seen as administratively less complex and time-consuming and more likely to produce a 'result' (see Whitney, 1994; OFSTED, 1995a; Rodgers, forthcoming).

The origins of 'Truancy Watch' lie in the conventional association between truancy and crime, the use of joint 'truancy sweeps' as a means of both improving school attendance and reducing juvenile crime recommended to LEAs and the police by the Elton Committee (DES, 1989a) and further endorsed by the DES in 1991 (DES, 1991b). LEA respondents to a national study conducted by Halford in 1991 indicated that over three quarters of LEAs had no involvement in truancy patrols (Halford, 1994). With explicit government encouragement the number of LEAs involved in 'Truancy Watch' programmes increased significantly by 1994–5 (Learmonth, 1995) although there was an equally significant decrease by 1996–7 (see below). Under such schemes, involving schools, the education welfare service, the police and the local business community, and sometimes social services and the youth service as well, central shopping areas are designated 'truancy-free' zones jointly patrolled by the police and education welfare officers. The introduction of schemes has usually been accompanied by a high-profile publicity and media campaign, often involving pupils themselves in designing publicity material, thus providing an awareness-raising opportunity within schools as well as encouraging pupil ownership of the value of attendance.

Despite concerns about risks to civil liberties associated with the ability of 'truancy patrols' to stop and question children and young people (Nowicka, 1993), 43 such projects were funded under the GEST initiative during 1994–5 (DFE, 1995c), rising to 45 in 1995–6 (DFEE, 1995c), although only 24 projects were being funded in 1996–7 (DFEE,

1996). An independent evaluation of 'Truancy Watch' schemes, commissioned by the Department for Education, concluded that there was little evidence of truants engaged in widespread criminal activity, that the police in some areas had insufficient resources to analyse data about juvenile crime committed in or around shopping areas during school hours, and the impact of schemes on 'hard core' truants was questionable, although the schemes had encouraged cooperation between individuals and organisations and had served to promote awareness within schools and more widely of the importance of school attendance (Learmonth, 1995).

While the longer-term impact of 'Truancy Watch' remains to be evaluated, Learmonth notes that resource shortages in police forces resulting in their inability to collect and analyse juvenile crime data mean that it is impossible to evaluate its impact on school-age offending linked to non-attendance. In the meantime the focus of many schemes has shifted from one which perceives the truant as a potential criminal to one which recognises their potential vulnerability, from missing out on education or as a victim of crime.

The way forward

General preventive measures can take place on a broad front: 'By far the largest deterrents to truancy are parental and teacher disapproval. . . . Greater teacher vigilance and closer school/home liaison might expand considerably on the figure of two thirds of pupils who do not truant' (O'Keeffe, 1994, p. 99).

One of the developments from the schools effectiveness research and increasing recognition of the role which schools themselves may play both in the creation and the resolution of difficulties which manifest themselves in school, has been the concept of the 'whole school' approach, although too few schools have developed this sufficiently systematically (Learmonth, 1995; OFSTED, 1995a). In keeping with the broad ethos of 'whole school' approaches a whole school attendance policy will ensure that the value of regular attendance permeates all aspects of school life, making the school a welcoming and positive environment for both teachers and pupils. It provides a framework which details clear and agreed procedures for dealing with absenteeism and ensures appropriate support for individual pupils with attendance problems. An effective whole school policy for attendance will also include provision for induction training for new staff and on-going training and development for all staff.

One of the first areas needing attention is the consistency of categorisation and registration of 'authorised' and 'unauthorised' absence and improvement in the accuracy of attendance registers. In some schools, under GEST initiatives (see below for further details), computerised registration schemes have been introduced which, while still reliant on the accuracy of information recorded, have the potential for improving the rigour and accessibility of attendance data, including enabling spot checks to be carried out speedily in individual lessons as a means of identifying prevalence and patterns of post-registration truancy. Computerised registration systems have proved effective in reducing staff time in data analysis, helping identify absence patterns and trends and determining appropriate interventions at individual, group or institutional level. For example, more accurate knowledge of absence patterns might not only reveal the absence levels of individual pupils or groups of pupils but might also highlight the vulnerability to absenteeism of particular lessons or teachers and consequently help determine the most efficient and effective forms and targets of intervention.

Whether or not a computerised registration system is installed, accurate registration will identify not only those pupils whose attendance is a cause of concern but also those with high levels of attendance. Increasing recognition has been given to the value of formal acknowledgement of good attendance at individual and group levels, such as the issue of certificates and letters to parents or carers and other tangible awards.

An effective 'whole school' policy will also ensure an equally prompt investigation and follow-up of absenteeism with both pupils and parents. In an efficient collaborative arrangement there will be agreement about the roles and responsibilities of different professionals, while investigation and follow-up of absence and the provision of support will not be delegated exclusively to the education welfare officer. In one inner-city high school, for example, pastoral staff initiated a telephone follow-up on the first day of all unexplained absence, considerably reducing the number of home visits which needed to be made. Pupils who have been absent from school for long periods as a result of illness or other authorised reason may often find returning difficult. The timely provision of appropriate support at this stage will usually minimise later problems and prevent the emergence of unauthorised absence. Improvements in the attendance of previously poor attenders – however slight – should also be formally acknowledged as a means of providing further encouragement to the individual pupil.

Increasingly, measures have been undertaken to anticipate the potential problems arising at secondary school transfer. Some LEAs have produced information leaflets such as 'Moving up to the Big School: What Every Year 6 Pupil Should Know' for all children about to transfer from primary school, and more efforts are generally being made to ensure as smooth a transfer as possible from primary to secondary schooling. Children with incipient attendance difficulties at primary school may be identified and supported individually during the transfer period and helped to establish regular attendance at secondary school.

Under the government's Grants for Education Support and Training (GEST) Programme a wide range of projects to improve school attendance and pupil behaviour have been established in England and

Wales since the early 1990s (and similar ventures encouraged in Northern Ireland and Scotland). The long-term effect of innovations promoted under these schemes has yet to be evaluated and, to date, dissemination of findings beyond the project schools and LEAs has been limited (Learmonth, 1995; Quality in Education Centre for Research and Consultancy, 1995; Kazi and Wilson, 1996).

A final comment we wish to make about a 'whole school' approach concerns the importance of the relationships between schools and external agencies and the fact that these are rarely unproblematic. With school attendance the relationship with the education welfare service is especially important. Potential problems focus on the precise nature of the education welfare officer's relationship with the school. On the one hand there is encouragement for the EWO to be seen as an integral member of the school team. For example, OFSTED (1995b) recognises the value of the EWO presence in school as indicated by their involvement in school-based training and other events and the provision of school-based facilities such as office space and access to a telephone. On the other hand the need for the EWO to be perceived as independent of the school is also important in work with pupils and families, in facilitating home–school links and acting a mediator or advocate. HMI's recognition that: 'Effective co-operation between the EWO and the school can improve attendance rates significantly, *especially when EWOs have concentrated on persuading schools to be more responsive to pupils' needs*' (DES, 1989b, p. vii – our emphasis), itself demands a relationship between EWO and school in which the EWO can exercise autonomy and authority and the school can tolerate tension.

CHAPTER 8

Disabled children

Introduction

This chapter provides an overview of models of disability and analyses the concepts of 'special educational need' and children 'in need'. It examines debates concerning 'integration' and 'segregation' and the role of the 'special education' system in marginalising and excluding certain groups of children and young people from mainstream education – and hence from wider society. Drawing on research of the 'special education' system, it will provide a focus on children and young people with physical disabilities and those with learning difficulties. Children with learning difficulties associated with emotional and behavioural difficulties are discussed separately in chapter 9. The relationship between (children with) 'special educational need' and (children) 'in need' is examined in terms of its implications for schools and social work agencies and requirements to establish cooperative arrangements.

Models of disability

Historically, legislation, policy and service provision for the disabled have been determined by a distinctive perspective on disability, variously described as the 'deficit', 'individual' or 'medical' model. It is a perspective which permeates our culture and is essentially one which devalues disabled people. It is evidenced in legislation which permits the termination of a pregnancy – in principle right up to the moment of birth – if there 'is a substantial risk that if the child were born it would suffer from such physical or mental abnormalities as to be seriously handicapped', and in perceptions of the birth of a disabled child as a 'tragic' event, following which parents are encouraged to mourn the loss of 'the child they really wanted' (Middleton, 1996). Parents who fail to respond to such encouragement risk further pathologisation by being seen as failing to 'accept' and 'come to terms' with their child's disability. Even if such perceptions are well-intentioned they serve to marginalise the disabled child and set them up for a lifetime of being 'second best'.

This model focuses on individual pathology in which the disabled person is seen as someone with a problem – and all-too-often results in the disabled individual being seen as a problem – because of their inability to engage in 'normal' activities or perform 'normal' social roles. Identification (diagnosis) of the disability by a variety of professional 'experts' – educational, medical, paramedical and social – leads to prognosis and the prescription of various 'treatments' designed to make the disabled person fit the demands of the non-disabled world, including medication, physical aids, physiotherapy, counselling/ psychotherapy and surgery. The failure of these measures to achieve the necessary 'fit' prompts the refinement of existing treatments and the search for new ones.

Another, and more insidious, consequence is that the disabled individual is seen as, at best, the passive victim of their disability (and becoming the involuntary recipient of others' pity or charity) or in some way contributing to their predicament and, at worst, excluded from mainstream society. As we show later in this chapter and in chapter 9, public and professional responses to disability are differentiated so that, while in educational terms both children with emotional and behavioural difficulties and physically disabled children might be regarded as having 'special educational needs', the former are more likely to be regarded as 'villains' and the latter as 'victims' and, therefore, more 'deserving'.

Disabled people may respond to the patronisation and hostility of non-disabled others in a variety of ways. Goffman (1968), in his pioneering work on 'stigma', claimed that the prime concern of those at risk of social stigma was to 'pass' themselves as 'normal'. Failing that (usually because the stigmatising condition or disability cannot be disguised) individuals attempt to minimise the significance of their condition by 'covering', for example, by reducing its visibility or by managing the disclosure of information about it. Conductive education, a controversial regime which aims to teach children with cerebral palsy motor skills to engage with others in as near 'normal' a way as possible, is a prime example of an attempt to 'normalise' physically disabled children, although at significant cost to both them and their families (Oliver, 1990) and, so far, without any tangible evidence of long-term benefit (Barstow *et al.*, 1993).

Goffman identifies a further strategy, 'withdrawal', which may be resorted to if 'passing' or 'covering' prove unsuccessful. While Goffman's analysis provides useful insights into social interactions surrounding disability, others (e.g. Morris, 1989, 1991) have challenged his preoccupation with the desire of the disabled to be seen as 'normal' (and the implicit assumption that they either accept or internalise the oppression of the non-disabled world) with the consequent limits this places on the options considered to be available to them.

Disabled people, for example, Finkelstein (1980, 1981) and Oliver (1983, 1990), have developed a 'social' model of disability as an empowering antidote to the dependency-enforcing deficit model. This model perceives disability not as the inability to meet 'normal' expectations, but as a barrier imposed by non-disabled individuals and social organisations which takes 'no or little account of people who have physical impairments and thus exclude(s) them from the mainstream of social activities' (UPIAS, 1976, p. 4). The physical, attitudinal and social barriers which prevent disabled individuals from securing full integration into mainstream society include poor employment prospects and consequent dependence on welfare benefits and/or charity; professional attitudes and services which patronise disabled people and encourage their dependency; inaccessible environments, and disabling experiences (e.g. care of disabled children which emphasises protection rather than promoting independence or encouraging social contact and perpetuates dependency into adulthood). The social model presents disability as an equal opportunities issue, emphasising the 'celebration of diversity' and the need for disabled children and adults to be valued and empowered, through the provision of necessary resources to 'ordinary' rather than 'special' services, to achieve participation in society on equal terms.

The male ideology which dominated the early social model, implying that the problems experienced by the disabled are exclusively socially constructed, has itself been challenged by disabled feminists such as Morris (1989, 1991). Advancing a more complete alternative social model Morris notes: 'A feminist perspective on disability must focus, not just on the socio-economic and ideological dimensions of our oppression, but also what it feels like to be unable to walk, to be in pain, to be incontinent, to have fits, to be unable to converse, to be blind or deaf, to have an intellectual ability which is much below the average' (Morris, 1991, p. 70).

Disability and 'special education'

The impact of the deficit model of disability in education has resulted in a focus on the individual child and the development of 'special' provision. Traditional assumptions both about the commitment, dedication, patience and altruism of those who work with disabled children and that looking after disabled children is more demanding than looking after non-disabled children have insulated much practice from criticism. However, there have been increasing concerns about the ideology, experience and outcomes of the 'special education' system, including separation, isolation, over-protection, low expectations, exclusion, unsuccessful integration and compulsory segregation.

The report of the Warnock Committee (HMSO, 1978) has set the scene for the provision of education for children with 'special educational needs' in Britain since the early 1980s, forming the basis of subsequent legislation. At the time the committee's recommendations were generally seen as a positive advance on previous thinking about, and provision for, disabled children. The committee proposed the abolition of the conventional distinction between 'non-handicapped' and 'handicapped' pupils (the latter including formal categorisation of forms of handicap) which had often led to unhelpful stereotyping and negative labelling without necessarily enhancing the education of disabled children. Instead the committee recommended that education provision should be based on identified 'special educational need'.

Drawing on a range of research studies the committee estimated that approximately one in six children at any one time and up to one in five at any time during their school careers would require some form of 'special educational provision', while a smaller group of pupils with significant disabilities (approximately 2 per cent of the total school population) should be formally assessed and issued with a statement of 'special educational need'.

Commensurate with the proposed abolition of the 'handicapped'/'non-handicapped' distinction, the committee suggested that most 'special education' provision should be met within mainstream schools with appropriate advisory and professional support. Nevertheless, despite the integrationist principles espoused by the committee, it identified a continuing role for special schools for children whose needs could not be met within mainstream schools or whose presence in mainstream schools would be too disruptive to the running of the school or to the educational progress of other pupils: those with 'severe or complex disabilities requiring specialist facilities, teaching methods or expertise'; those with 'severe' emotional, behavioural or relationship difficulties, and those who fail to make progress in mainstream school despite additional support who are 'more likely to thrive in the more intimate communal and educational setting of a special school' (HMSO, 1978, p. 96).

The limits of the 'special education' system

Following the Warnock Committee's recommendations a child is considered to have 'special educational needs' if they have a learning difficulty which calls for 'special educational provision' to be made for them. A child has a 'learning difficulty' if they:

- have a significantly greater difficulty in learning than the majority of children of the same age;
- have a disability which either prevents or hinders them from making use of educational facilities of a kind generally provided for children of their age in schools within the area of the education authority concerned, or
- are under the age of five years and are, or would be if 'special educational provision' was not made for them, likely to meet either of the two criteria outlined above.

'Special education' is defined as education provision which is additional to, or otherwise different from, the educational provision made generally for children of the same age in maintained schools, other than special schools.

The general duty to provide appropriate education within mainstream school, wherever possible, for children with 'special educational needs' was qualified by the requirements to take account of the wishes of the child's parents, and to ensure the 'efficient use of resources' and the 'efficient education' of other children.

With hindsight the failure of integration (the proportion of the total school population attending special schools – approximately 1.3 per cent – remaining constant (DES, 1990; Weddell, 1993)) should not be surprising. Barnes, for example, criticises the Warnock Committee for failing to challenge traditional perceptions of disability or conventional wisdom regarding the education of disabled children: 'While the demedicalisation of the labelling of disabled individuals within the educational context must be viewed positively ... it represents little more than a cosmetic exercise.... The emphasis is still on the inadequacy of the individual: it is s/he who is different; it is s/he who is at fault; and, most importantly, it is s/he who must change' (Barnes, 1994, p. 33), a view of education which is hardly compatible with the right of disabled children to enjoy a 'full and decent life, in conditions which ensure dignity, promote self-reliance, and facilitate the child's active participation in the community' (UN Convention on the Rights of the Child, 1989, Article 23).

More fundamentally, Tomlinson (1981, 1982) analyses the role of 'special education' and 'special schools' as primarily instruments of social control which ensure the efficiency and smooth functioning of mainstream education through the removal of 'troublesome' children, in particular focusing on children with learning difficulties. As we show in chapter 9, the removal from mainstream education of children with emotional and behavioural difficulties may have a similar effect.

The specific failings of the 'special education' system can be located at both individual school and LEA level. Within mainstream schools there is generally limited physical access for disabled pupils and, by implication, for other disabled people such as parents. For example, a report by HMI which focused on mainstream secondary schools where an attempt had been made to integrate physically disabled pupils noted poor physical accommodation, access and resources: 'Difficulties include inadequate storage space, particularly for wheelchairs and other large equipment; inappropriate safe provision for the charging of batteries for electric wheelchairs; too small hygiene and toileting provision that limits wheelchair access; inappropriate furniture for changing children in privacy; poor disposal facilities for soiled material; and inappropriate and inaccessible facilities' (DES, 1989c, p. 11). The same report notes that mainstream schools do not always provide an appropriate experience for their disabled pupils, recording the frequently wide gap between recognition of the principle of endorsing disabled children's independence and actively promoting it.

And this represents, if not 'best' practice, at least 'better-than-worst' practice for, as Barnes (1994) comments, health and safety regulations are often presented by schools as reasons for not admitting disabled pupils in the first place. Another HMI report (DES 1989d) observes that some mainstream schools did not have properly adapted toilets and changing facilities for non-ambulant and incontinent pupils. While the lack of resources and their efficient utilisation will often be used to justify the lack of provision and accessibility, in many instances the cost of adaptations to improve accessibility would not necessarily be high (Coopers and Lybrand, 1993) and, given the market analogy, we should not overlook the fact that supermarkets manage to provide such facilities as a matter of course!

More seriously (echoing Tomlinson's critique) there is evidence of discrimination against pupils with 'special educational needs' within the mainstream sector. An HMI report of provision in mainstream schools for primary-aged children with 'special educational needs' (DES, 1989d) notes that such pupils were not wholly accepted by teachers in a number of schools. The extent of institutional discrimination within the mainstream sector adds weight to those who would argue for the maintenance and development of segregated provision as being better than placement in an environment which continually marginalises disabled children. This view sees the provision of decent specialist services as an essential step towards genuine integration in society. Since 'special schools' are better placed to provide the education needed, 'special provision' is a form of positive action which provides disabled children 'a better start in life' (Simpson, 1990).

However, the quality of accommodation and resources in special schools has been criticised by HMI – at best 'satisfactory', at worst 'downright dangerous' (DES 1989c–e). In addition, despite claims that reintegration of pupils into mainstream education is a principal aim of such schools, this is frequently frustrated by the failure to teach a curriculum commensurate with that taught in local mainstream schools. Small schools, in particular, have difficulty in providing a full range of necessary facilities (DES, 1989e). O'Reilly (1996b) claims that up to a third of special schools fail to meet official standards or have serious weaknesses. Barnes finds little evidence of the beneficial effect of special schools which he describes as: 'a fundamental part of the discriminatory process, not simply because they create and perpetuate artificial barriers between disabled children and their non-disabled peers, but also because they reinforce traditional individualistic medical perceptions of disability, and generally, fail to provide their pupils with either an adequate education or the skills necessary for adulthood' (Barnes, 1994, p. 42).

Assessment and statementing procedures have also been criticised. Examination of the operation of the 1981 Education Act by the House of Commons Education Committee (1993) and the Audit Commission and HMI (1992) found confusion about what constitutes 'special educational needs' and the respective responsibilities of LEAs, schools and other agencies to meet them; a lack of clear accountability by schools and LEAs for the progress made by pupils at the earlier stages of assessment and for the resources received to meet children's 'special educational needs', and wide variations and inconsistencies between

LEAs as to which children were provided with statements and a lack of clarity about different levels of need. These conclusions have been reinforced by other studies. For example, Meltzer, Smyth and Robus (1989) produce evidence of disabled children being placed in 'special schools' *without* a statement (Grimshaw and Berridge (1994) identifying similar practices in their study of children with emotional and behavioural difficulties). Rogers (1986) found that most LEAs failed to provide details about sources of support and advice to parents; half failed to give parents adequate information on the assessment and statutory procedures under the 1981 Education Act; only a third told parents they had a right to be fully consulted and to receive all relevant information and almost half did not give information on appeals arrangements.

The length of time taken to complete the formal assessment and statementing process is subject to considerable delay and variation between LEAs, in extreme cases up to three years (Audit Commission and HMI, 1992; RADAR, 1992). In some instances delay and slowing down the assessment and statementing process may be a deliberate strategy on the part of an LEA to save stretched resources (Hagedorn, 1992), while other LEAs have been placed under further pressure as the result of major increases in referrals from schools seeking additional resources to support individual children or to excuse poor 'league table' performance (Lee, 1990; Pyke 1990; Croall, 1991). Empirical evidence of the increased demand on LEA resources is provided in a report from auditors Coopers and Lybrand (unpublished at the time of writing) recording a two thirds increase in the numbers of pupils with statements of 'special educational need' (cited in Pyke, 1996).

'Special educational needs' and education reform

Concerns about the philosophy and quality of 'special education' did not feature high in the agenda for education reforms promoted by the Education Reform Act 1988 and subsequent legislation (see chapter 3). Indeed, for many commentators, the introduction of the education market, the changing roles of, and relationships between, schools and LEAs, and the increased bureaucratic pressures associated with the introduction of the National Curriculum, resulting from the educational reforms have not best served the interests of children with 'special educational needs'.

In particular, the principle of integration of children with 'special educational needs' has been severely undermined. Head teachers may be even less willing than before to admit − or keep − disabled children who may have a negative impact on the school's performance statistics or its image. Additionally the impact of delegation of funding under LMS or DSM might make schools more reluctant to purchase support services (previously provided free by the LEA) for individual pupils and consequently less willing to accept in the first place pupils needing such services (Coopers and Lybrand Deloitte, 1988), while the reducing proportion of education resources retained within LEAs means that their scope for providing support services is much reduced. As we observe in chapter 9, some head teachers find it easier to exclude children who may have a statement of 'special educational need' or who may be awaiting assessment than provide the additional support or resources required to maintain the child in a mainstream placement. The consequent scenario, highlighted by Whitty and Menter (1991), is that the new hierarchy of schools, driven by market pressures and formula funding, will result in children with 'special educational needs' being concentrated in schools which otherwise experience recruitment difficulties. For example, one of the significant pressures facing the Ridings School in Halifax in an area where the most academically able pupils were 'creamed off' by local grant-maintained schools was claimed to be the exceptionally high proportion of pupils in the school with 'special educational needs' (BBC, 1996).

Perhaps even more insidious is that while the 'special education' system makes no claim to being a 'rights-based' service, it can hardly be judged to be a 'needs-led' one either as evidence has emerged of assessments and statements being framed to utilise available resources rather than addressing the individual needs of children (e.g. Berliner, 1990; Hofkins, 1990). These shortcomings have led Baroness Warnock to argue that: 'the whole concept of "statementing" for only a few children with the rest supposedly having their needs met according to what individual schools can provide, must be radically rethought' (Warnock, 1992).

Against this backdrop the government introduced the Education Act 1993 which, although primarily concerned with extending the role of the education market, together with the accompanying Code of Practice on the Identification and Assessment of 'special educational needs' (DFE, 1994b) addresses issues of 'special educational needs' and some of the specific shortcomings of the system which we have highlighted earlier. The Act defines more precisely schools' responsibilities towards children who have 'special educational needs' by requiring them to produce a 'special educational needs' policy (including information about the school's 'special educational' provision; its policies for identification, assessment and provision for pupils with 'special educational needs'; and staffing policies and partnerships with external bodies) and to report annually to parents on its implementation. The Act also increases the rights of parents to express a preference for particular schools; prescribes time limits within which assessment should take place; and streamlines procedures for appeal against assessments and provision.

In addition, the Code of Practice provides practical guidance to schools and LEAs on how to meet their respective responsibilities to children with 'special educational needs', emphasising the importance of early identification and assessment of 'special educational needs' and the importance of a range of partnerships (involving parents, education and other agencies) in finding the best way to meet these; the need for a systematic approach to assessment, and ensuring that all pupils with 'special educational needs' 'have the greatest possible access to a broad and balanced education' which includes the National Curriculum. In recognition that the majority of children with 'special educational needs' are in mainstream schools, both the Act and Code of Practice re-state the principle of integration, 'where appropriate and taking account of the wishes of their parents'. Baroness Warnock, among others, was not convinced that the 1993 Act would represent much of a new deal for children with 'special educational needs': 'the drawback with such amendments is that they will be introduced against the background of the old ill-drawn line between those who do and those who do not merit statements. What happens to those whose needs still exist, but for whom the education authority has no statutory duty remains untouched. The suspicion must be that these children will be increasingly pushed to one side' (Warnock, 1992).

The Disability Discrimination Act 1995 (and broadly parallel legislation in Northern Ireland and Scotland) provides few additional safeguards for disabled pupils, restating existing general obligations regarding integrated education and schools' duties to produce and publish a 'special needs' policy together with information about their provision for disabled pupils. The Act does not require schools to improve access to facilities. The Act is generally weaker than its sex and race discrimination counterparts and does not provide a legally enforceable individual right to an integrated education.

The social model of disability and inclusive education

There is a danger that responses to the 1993 Act and the Code of Practice could mean no more than mechanistic lip-service to the specific issues identified in the Regulations which might espouse the language, but not necessarily the spirit, of equal opportunities. The second major danger is the privatisation of policies and practices which are informed and owned only by those in the school with recognised 'expertise' in, or responsibility for, 'special educational needs', rather than the development of whole school policies and approaches. What must not be overlooked, despite the survival of a significant segregated 'special education' sector, is that not only are the majority of children with identified 'special educational needs' in mainstream schools, the typical non-selective school will always contain pupils across the spectrum of physical and intellectual ability, as well as pupils formally diagnosed as having 'special education needs'. Such recognition emphasises the dangers of creating artificial distinctions not only between children with 'special educational needs' in 'special schools' and those with 'special educational needs' in mainstream schools, but also between those pupils in mainstream schools who have identified 'special educational needs' and those who don't, and challenges mainstream schools to provide adequate provision for all their pupils.

The social model of disability helps us to move beyond the concept of integration (poorly implemented though this still is) to the more demanding – and ultimately more productive concept of inclusion.

Inclusive education means more than pupils with different abilities and characteristics being in the same school or in the same class. The Council for Disabled Children (1994) has defined inclusion as: 'a philosophy which views diversity of strengths, abilities and needs as natural and desirable, bringing to any community the opportunity to respond in ways which lead to learning and growth for the whole school community and giving each and every member a valued role. Inclusion requires striving for the optimal growth of all pupils in the most enabling environment by recognising individual strengths and needs' (cited in Russell, 1995, p. 20).

The Centre for Studies on Inclusive Education, identifying 'ten reasons for inclusion', regards inclusive education as a 'human right', 'good education' and 'good social sense':

' 1 All children have a right to learn together.
2 Children should not be devalued or discriminated against by being excluded or sent away because of their disability or learning difficulty.
3 Children do not need to be protected from each other. Disabled adults, describing themselves as special school survivors, are now demanding an end to segregation.
4 There are no legitimate reasons to separate children for their education. Children belong together with advantages and benefits for everyone.
5 Research shows children do better academically and socially in integrated settings.
6 There is no teaching or care in a segregated school which cannot take place in an ordinary school.
7 Given commitment and support, inclusive education is a more efficient use of educational resources.
8 Segregation teaches children to be fearful, ignorant and breeds prejudice.
9 All children need an education that will help them develop relationships and prepare them for life in the mainstream.
10 Only inclusion has the potential to reduce fear and to build friendship, respect and understanding' (cited in Middleton, 1996, p. 45).'

In practice inclusion means a commitment by the entire school community to overcome all physical, social and attitudinal barriers preventing the participation of disabled children and adults in school life on equal terms with the non-disabled. Clearly attitudes are as important as resources – if not more so – and inclusion cannot be successfully achieved without the development of disability awareness and equality training opportunities. Inclusion does not mean that pupils and schools can – or should be expected to – manage without specialist support. Inclusion does mean ensuring that school buildings and facilities are accessible to both disabled pupils and to disabled parents (Coopers and Lybrand, 1993; see also chapter 6 for issues relating to disabled parents and access to schools).

Practical steps which schools can take to increase awareness of disability and increase the participation of disabled people in school life include imaginative use of computer technology and the National Curriculum and the development of school behaviour policies. The increased participation in mainstream schools of pupils with sensory and physical impairments and those with communications and learning difficulties can be facilitated by the use of computers and information technology, as well as dedicated computer-assisted learning and communications. Such equipment is becoming more widely available in all mainstream schools, often with the 'support of supermarket chains' (Blyth and Milner, 1996d). Rieser (1995) identifies ways in which the National Curriculum can provide ideas for the whole school curriculum and disability policies. This can include opening up debates about disability and the way it is presented in language, literature, the media and the visual arts. Science and geography can provide the basis for developing understanding of the causes of impairment, while the PSE curriculum provides opportunities for raising debate about the social causes of disability and responses to it.

Rieser also highlights the value of whole school behaviour policies in promoting the inclusion of disabled pupils by mediating boisterous behaviour which can intimidate and exclude some disabled children, especially in locations outside the classroom. Such policies can emphasise respect for others and – despite a prevailing contrary culture within education as a whole – an ethos of collaboration rather than competition.

Rieser argues that all pupils (and staff) benefit from a commitment to inclusion. Inclusive policies and practices respect and value individual differences and recognise that we all have a variety of abilities. Learning and living alongside others who may be quite different will help to dispel the fears and unfamiliarity which lead to prejudice and discrimination, encouraged by exclusion and segregation. This analysis suggests that the statutory requirement that integration of disabled pupils into mainstream schools should not conflict with the interests of other pupils should be interpreted broadly. Rather than discounting inclusion on the grounds of additional expense, inconvenience or the need to change customary practices, serious account should be taken of the long-term costs of *not* pursuing inclusion.

Social work, disabled children and the Children Act 1989

Consideration of provision for disabled children would not be complete without discussion of the Children Act which provides the central legislative framework in England and Wales for the provision of services for disabled children. The Act places on local authorities a duty to:

* minimise the effect of disability on disabled children within their area, and
* give disabled children the opportunity to 'lead lives which are as normal as possible' i.e. focusing on providing assistance in partnership with the child's normal carers (Children Act 1989, Schedule 2, para. 6).

A major concept under the Act is that of children 'in need'. In chapter 6 we have already outlined the first and second limbs of the definition of 'in need' under Section 17 and Schedule 2 of the Act. A child is also considered to be 'in need' if they are disabled. Controversially the Act retains anachronistic definitions of disability, derived from the deficit model, ostensibly to ensure consistency with existing legislation (i.e. a person is disabled who is 'blind, deaf or dumb or who suffer(s) from mental disorder of any description' or who is 'substantially and permanently handicapped by illness, injury, or congenital deformity or such other disabilities as may be prescribed'). However, this ignores the fact that such consistency could have been achieved had the opportunity been taken to revise and overhaul the legislative framework governing provision for the disabled. The Act's conceptualisation that disabled children are: 'less capable and require placing in a distinctive category ("children in need") transmits negative messages to society, parents and children; even to abusers. It does not say "these children are powerful and valuable", but suggests they are weak and incapable of independence. . . . Disabled children have been taught to be good victims' (Kennedy, 1995, p. 149).

In similar vein Kennedy argues that the Act's requirement that local authorities keep a register of children with disabilities is a prejudicial and discriminatory act to which no other category of children is subjected.

Nevertheless, designation as being 'in need' is a passport to services under the Act, which places a duty on local authorities to identify children 'in need' in their locality and to provide and publicise information about any services which might help them. (See chapter 6 for a summary of local authority services for children 'in need'.) The broad definition of 'in need' under the Act is deliberate, giving local authorities considerable discretion in identifying the extent of local need and prioritising services in the context of identified need, statutory responsibilities and resources available. The Act itself does little to ensure the resourcing of adequate services, as illustrated by a study conducted by the Department of Health Social Services Inspectorate of services to disabled children and their families in four local authority areas: 'All four authorities intended to provide a range of services designed to minimise the effect of disability on the disabled child. The extent to which they achieved this intention was hampered by the sizeable mis-match between the resources provided and the demand for services. Many parents were unable to get access to the support they required in order to continue caring for their child until they reached crisis point' (SSI, 1994, p. 5).

Because of the different definitions used to categorise 'special educational need' and 'in need' a child with 'special educational need' may or may not also be regarded by the local authority as a child 'in need'. Similarly a child may be considered to be 'in need' yet not have a recognised 'special educational need'. The importance of local authority discretion to determine whether certain groups of children are to be considered to be 'in need' and the consequent extent to which the accident of geographical location affects access to appropriate services is illustrated by evaluation of the first year of implementation of the Children Act in England (HMSO, 1993). Under the first limb of the definition of 'in need' approximately half of the local authorities providing information (27) included children with 'special educational needs'. What is clearly significant about these findings is the proportion of local authorities which did *not* consider this group of children to be 'in need'. In addition it might be reasonably supposed that the overall proportion of local authorities not including children with 'special educational needs' within the 'in need' definition could be higher since the 45 per cent of English local authorities which did not provide information for this study is more likely to have included those which had not been proactive in implementing the Act.

Oliver (1983) identifies three key skills which social workers have to offer disabled children and their families: provision of emotional support; access to relevant practical assistance, and reduction of the negative impact of having to deal with discriminatory organisations and bureaucracies. Middleton (1996) argues that social workers must value the individual rights of disabled children, adopting a 'children first' approach. She also sees social workers as providing: accurate inform-ation (including the benefits system and other sources of financial help; details of solicitors who are competent in establishing trust funds; the child's and parents' legal rights; local support groups) and acting as agents of change alongside the child and parents, providing advocacy and promotion of self-advocacy. Middleton also argues that, in their role as care managers, social workers (and other social services staff) need to ensure that the services they are accessing on behalf of the child (such as educational, medical and care facilities) are non-discriminatory and safe. This is especially important given that educational, health and care settings have often provided opportunities for the abuse of disabled children, an issue we discuss in more detail in chapter 10.

The Children Act provides a framework for partnership and collaborative arrangements for assessment and provision of services involving statutory and voluntary health, education and welfare agencies, children and parents, Section 27 of the Act and Section 166 of the Education Act 1993 imposing reciprocal (but qualified) duties to co-operate across education, social services and health agency boundaries.

However, as a result of changing and increasing responsibilities, insufficient resources and agency reorganisation, there is little evidence of the establishment of effective inter agency or interdisciplinary services for children (e.g. Audit Commission and HMI, 1992; Audit Commission, 1994; Grimshaw and Berridge, 1994; Sinclair, 1994; Sinclair *et al.*, 1994; SSI, 1994; SSI and OFSTED, 1995).

The obligation on social workers to operate within the legislative context, agency boundaries and resources is clearly a limiting factor for practice. Nevertheless, despite the overwhelming picture of inadequate and oppressive service provision for disabled children, the (albeit isolated) examples of good practice (e.g. SSI, 1994) and evidence of innovative developments of inclusive education (e.g. Rieser, 1995; Russell, 1995) indicate the extent to which positive change is possible, despite resource limitations and less-than-helpful legislation.

CHAPTER 9

Pupils with behaviour problems

Introduction

Children's behaviour problems have always been of concern to adults whether these consist of young children's challenges to parental authority or youth *per se* being seen as a potential threat to the stability and order of society more generally. Given the relationship between education and wider society, pupils' behaviour problems contain the potential to reflect anxieties about families' abilities to socialise their children effectively and schools' abilities to prepare children for the world of work and adult citizenship. There is intense concern, therefore, to deal with pupil behaviour problems swiftly before they become sustained challenges to wider social rules and challenging behaviour is viewed most seriously when it is exhibited by pupils occupying the transitional position between childhood and adulthood. This position is not fixed, being defined differently depending upon the age at which children enter the workforce. For example, Flora Thompson, in *Lark Rise to Candleford*, comments: 'It must be remembered that in those days a boy of eleven was nearing the end of his school life. Soon he would be at work, already he felt himself almost a man and too old for petticoat government. However, those were country boys, wild and rough, and many of them were as tall as she [the teacher] was. Those who failed to pass Standard IV and so could not leave school until they were eleven looked upon that last year as a punishment inflicted upon them by the school authorities and behaved accordingly' (Thompson, 1945, p. 182).

Changing perceptions of pupil behaviour problems

Disaffection with schooling provided the dominant explanation of pupil behaviour problems in the 1970s, being largely considered an active response on the part of low-achieving pupils who did not see school as relevant to their future careers (see, for example, Willis, 1977). Other studies (e.g. HMI, 1978a, b; Hughes, 1984) also identified bored, failing pupils as those most likely to be disaffected with schooling even though many such pupils reacted with patience and resignation rather than hostility (HMI, 1979). Claxton (1984) went somewhat further, indicating that pupil behaviour problems were located in a deep dissatisfaction with schooling which provided not only a monumental irrelevance to pupils' lives but was also a deeply humiliating experience.

Generally, a number of studies agreed that pupil disaffection with schooling was largely rational and reasonable (for an overview, see Furlong, 1991). The extent of violent and disruptive behaviour in schools was relatively low (for an overview, see Hart, 1977) and links between juvenile delinquency and pupil disaffection were far from straightforward (e.g. Carlen, 1987; Graham and Bowling, 1995).

The prescribed remedies tended to be largely individual and specialist. Pastoral care developed rapidly at this time with an emphasis on counselling, withdrawal and nurture groups (see, for example, Scottish Office Education Department, 1977; HMI, 1978a, b). Where these methods did not yield results, pupils were transferred to off-site behavioural units where it was hoped that 'the work of the units should make it possible to identify effective and successful practice' (HMI, 1978b, p. 42). However, despite the advantageous staff:pupil ratios the quality of education left much to be desired and the success of units was questionable (e.g. Mongon, 1988; Cooper *et al.*, 1991; ACE, 1992): 'Units and their pupils occupy an ambiguous legal twilight zone and, although this offers some freedom to manoeuvre and the ability to be flexible, children are poorly served' (OFSTED, 1993a, p. 9).

Noting that few pupils ever returned to mainstream schooling, and the implications of this for their longer-term futures, Tomlinson (1981, 1982) was even more scathing of the effect of 'special education' in marginalising certain groups of pupils.

Disillusionment with the results of behavioural units triggered the beginning of a preoccupation with another explanation of pupil behaviour problems which increasingly became labelled as 'disruptive behaviour' rather than 'disaffection'. Despite this term perhaps indicating more pupil responsibility for the behaviour, the focus generally shifted from the individual pupil to the school, boosted by a series of studies in the 1980s which demonstrated that schools with good examination results and attendance patterns also had significantly fewer pupil behaviour problems than less successful schools, regardless of intake, and which we have reviewed in chapter 2.

Positive behaviour programmes became the accepted way not only to 'cure behaviour problems' but also to ensure that they were prevented from occurring in the first place. However, attempts to explain behaviour problems in terms of teacher insensitivity to pupil problems or whole school failings did not survive the 1990s' preoccupation with 'dangerous' and 'delinquent' children.

It was no longer possible simply to talk about pupil behaviour problems when children's crime ranged from murder, rape and mugging to joy-riding, theft and vandalism. The sheer extent of the violence and the recidivist nature of much of the more 'minor' crime meant that children's accounts could not be 'recycled' to provide a therapy rather than a punishment frame as had happened previously (Aronsson, 1991). The media and public identified a hard core of recidivist and dangerous children, particularly boys aged between ten and thirteen, and blamed unruly, lone-parent families and a drug/video culture rather than inadequate discipline in schools. Teachers, however, defined dangerous children rather more widely and distanced themselves from responsibility for the behaviour; pupil behaviour problems were to be seen as part of the ills of society, not a failure of school discipline or teacher engagement with low-achieving pupils.

Teachers did this by two processes. First, they joined the public bandwagon of concern about children's violence, casting themselves and well-behaved pupils as victims. Teacher reports of pupil violence became commonplace. For example, the 1994 NAS/UWT annual conference detailed a catalogue of bullying, extortion, intimidation, vandalism, swearing, racism and sexism as everyday occurrences among pupils bored with lessons. Vice-president Peter Cole told conference delegates: 'Unless there is a redressing of the balance and a genuine development of a supportive partnership, then there is a real prospect of schools moving towards anarchy' (*Yorkshire Post*, 1994). Thus, school was not presented as a subsystem of the socialisation process which was failing but as being unduly influenced in its main task by failures in other subsystems which might cause its collapse. Second, schools promoted the idea that rather than presenting a challenge to their teaching expertise, pupils with problems were actually a threat to the largely well-behaved body of pupils, thus changing the emphasis from a few disruptive pupils to disrupted lessons. This was entirely understandable as testing meant that teachers were concentrating on middle-range pupils, as a result of the need to bring a GCSE D grade pupil into the important A–C grades to improve overall school performance, and was guaranteed to be popular with a large number of parents. It had the effect of reducing teacher incentives to spend time with low-achieving pupils as school performance was measured by results rather than progress. Thus, teachers began to distance themselves from low-achieving pupils and the emphasis of positive behaviour policies shifted. Tackling bullying, vandalism, drug taking etc. became issues to do with providing a school atmosphere in which the majority of pupils would not have their lessons disrupted by a minority of dangerous pupils. At the same time, psychological and social work support services for schools were reduced and budgets rarely allowed for the buying-in of specialist services. Pupils with behaviour problems became undesirable 'commodities' for schools (for a fuller discussion, see Blyth and Milner, 1996d).

Exclusion from school

The result is that since the early 1990s there has been an inexorable growth in the numbers of pupils excluded from school (e.g. DFE, 1992c; Gardiner, 1996), such practice being contrary to the ostensible spirit of integration espoused within policies towards 'special educational needs'

(Garner, 1996). (For an overview of exclusion policy and practice see Blyth and Milner, 1996b.) However, close analysis of the available data helps to expose myths about the prevalence of unacceptable behaviour, especially violence, in British schools.

Despite the significant rise in the numbers of recorded exclusions, less than one fifth of one per cent of pupils in English schools are perma- nently excluded, although certain groups of pupils are more exposed to the risk of exclusion than others, in particular: boys; African-Caribbeans – especially boys; children with low levels of academic attainment; children in public care; children from disadvantaged socio-economic backgrounds, and children with 'special educational needs'. These groups are not, of course, mutually exclusive. The link between exclusion and 'special educational needs' is one which has received little attention to date. OFSTED has acknowledged the existence of a 'hard core of pupils with whom it is unrealistic to expect mainstream schools to cope' the severity of whose emotional and behavioural difficulties constitute a 'special educational need', but which is fre-quently overlooked prior to exclusion (OFSTED, 1996b, p. 29). The government itself recognises that the concept of emotional and behavioural difficulties embraces a continuum of pupil behaviour ranging from naughtiness and disruption which is both 'normal' and 'unacceptable' to behaviour which may be symptomatic of serious underlying mental illness (DFE and DOH, 1994a). Physical assault on staff by pupils invariably results in permanent exclusion, yet exclusion for violent behaviour remains at a relatively low level (DFE, 1992c; NUT, 1992; Imich, 1994; OFSTED, 1996b). Most exclusions do not result from 'one-off' serious incidents, but from cumulative 'disobedience' (DFE, 1993) – a constellation of negative, disruptive, insolent and uncooperative behaviours (NUT, 1992; DFE, 1993, OFSTED, 1996b). In many instances the event precipitating exclusion may be relatively trivial, but providing the 'final straw' for a deteriorating pupil/teacher relationship.

It is, nevertheless, true that official statistics mask the true rate of exclusions (although it is unlikely that the extent of serious physical violence in schools is significantly under-reported). Schools are not obliged to notify LEAs of fixed-term exclusions so available data about these is likely to be incomplete. In addition there is evidence of schools resorting to various forms of 'unofficial', 'informal' or 'internal' exclu-sion, the prevalence of which, for obvious reasons, has been difficult to calculate. Examples include inappropriate authorisation of study leave (OFSTED, 1995a) and sending home pupils because of 'inappropriate' clothing (Knight, 1996; Stirling, 1996) or for spurious health reasons (Stirling, 1996), and encouraging parents to 'voluntarily withdraw' the pupil and secure a place for them in another school (SHA, 1992). Similar practices occur in Scotland, where some Education Authorities permit unofficial 'cooling off' periods without the pupil being formally excluded (Cullen, 1996).

Inevitably global statistics mask other trends, such as the considerable variations between schools' exclusion rates and practi OFSTED (1996b) considers 'unacceptable' the differences betwe some schools being 'irresponsibly profligate' in their recourse t exclusion and others placing staff and other pupils at risk by not excluding soon enough. Suggestions that these differences can be largely, if not exclusively, explained by the nature of schools' intakes (SHA, 1992) have been discounted by the government (DFE, 1992c). OFSTED (1996b) identifies a link between schools with high rates of exclusion serving catchments with high levels of socio-economic deprivation, while also providing evidence of low excluding and 'well behaved' schools serving similarly disadvantaged areas. It therefore favours explanations for school variation in exclusions which focus on differences in school policies and attitudes towards behaviour and schools' differential ability to prevent behaviour which might result in exclusion from occurring in the first place. Geographical variation in exclusion rates, largely the result of education authority policies, has also been noted in Scotland (Cullen, 1996). Given the evidence reviewed in chapter 2, it is highly likely that both school processes and contextual factors relating to the social and economic environment in which schools operate contribute to differences in exclusion levels at individual schools.

Explanations for the rise in exclusions also need to be sought at different levels. We provide a summary of these below. More detailed discussion may be found in Rutter (1991b); NUT (1992); SHA (1992); Parsons *et al.* (1995); Blyth and Milner (1996b); OFSTED (1996b); Stirling (1996).

Within schools the rise in exclusions – and increased reluctance of schools to admit pupils excluded from another school – has been attributed to the effects of education reforms including: additional administrative workloads on teachers resulting in higher levels of stress (and less tolerance of threats to manageable working conditions) and less time for pastoral matters; pressures to improve standards and schools' images; increasing financial and administrative independence of schools from LEAs; increased competition (and decreased cooperation) between schools, and reduced LEA support services. In addition school behaviour policies may expedite pupils' progress through the tariff system towards early exclusion. External factors which have been cited include: deteriorating home circumstances and lack of parental discipline; increases in family poverty and socio-economic disadvantage; and increases in various forms of child psychiatric disorder. In particular there has been increasing interest in the phenomenon of Attention Deficit Disorder (ADD) or Attention Deficit Hyperactivity Disorder (ADHD). It is claimed that upwards of 5 per cent of school-age children may be affected by attention deficit disorders, behavioural conditions which are caused by an imbalance of neurological chemical transmitters. Recognised treatment is primarily by medication (usually amphetamines), supplemented with psychological, behavioural and cognitive-behavioural interventions in the home and school (Barkley,

1990). Since the existence of attention deficit disorders is based on the assessment of behavioural symptoms rather than a direct test for neuro-chemical deficiency, diagnosis and treatment remain controversial. For example, in a survey of ten and eleven year olds, Schachar *et al.* (1981) found little consistency in symptom identification between parents and teachers. Although teachers identified 8.3 per cent of the children as hyperactive and the parents identified 9.9 per cent, only 2.2 per cent of the children were rated as hyperactive by both teachers and parents.

The consequences of exclusion

Despite formal provisions for appeals and review of exclusions decisions, exclusions are rarely challenged by parents, local education authorities or school governing bodies. Where parents do exercise their right of appeal against their child's exclusion their chances of success are slim indeed (DFE, 1993) and a case has been made that judicial review might better serve the interests of pupils and their parents (Allen, 1994). Nevertheless, at least some educational professionals perceive existing rights of appeal against exclusion as a threat to the maintenance of school discipline and the authority of teachers, even contemplating strike action in the face of (rare) governors' decisions to overturn a head teacher's decision to permanently exclude a pupil.

For most pupils, therefore, permanent exclusion is unlikely to be reversed, and as a result they are exposed to serious educational and other social consequences. As we have indicated, the likelihood of permanently excluded pupils being offered a place in another mainstream school is increasingly unlikely (NUT, 1992; SHA, 1992; OFSTED, 1996b), Parsons *et al.* (1995) observing that, nationally, only 15 per cent of pupils excluded from secondary school return to mainstream school. In any event there will often be considerable delay in providing any alternative form of education (DFE, 1992c; Mitchell, 1996). Some young people may reach school-leaving age while still excluded (Hackett, 1992) and others completely disappear from the world of formal education (SHA, 1992). Home tuition is a common type of provision – and more so for excluded primary school pupils – although it is rarely provided at a level which equates with 'full-time' education (Parsons *et al.*, 1995).

In the light of the widespread concerns about education provision for excluded pupils the government proposed the revival of behavioural units (many of which had closed because of financial cutbacks) in the guise of Pupil Referral Units. Initial evidence of the performance of PRUs is mixed, although a longer-term evaluation will be necessary to establish whether they will be able to overcome the shortcomings of their forebears. As it is, few appear to be working satisfactorily (OFSTED, 1995c; Parsons *et al.*, 1995), although Parsons *et al.* (1995), Fisher (1996) and Normington (1996) indicate the scope for PRUs to make a positive contribution to the education of excluded pupils. Since the annual cost of off-site provision was approximately £7,000 per pupil in 1993 (OFSTED, 1993a) – about three times the cost of educating a pupil in a mainstream school – evaluation of the quality of PRU provision needs to take account of what a mainstream school could provide given a similar level of resources – or a Cities in Schools 'Bridge Project' costing between £4,000 and £4,500 per pupil per year (Stephenson, 1996).

While the major tangible costs of exclusion fall on education authorities, these are not the only costs of exclusion. There is increasing concern that excluded children may become involved in delinquency (see, for example, DFE, 1993; AMA, 1995; Condon, 1995; Graham and Bowling, 1995; Audit Commission, 1996b; Cullingford and Morrison, 1996). As a corollary the National Association for the Care and Resettlement of Offenders (1997) has highlighted the potential crime-prevention role of schools through integrating the least able and most disaffected pupils and reducing exclusions. Consequently social services and the criminal justice system may also incur costs as a result of exclusion (Parsons *et al.*, 1994; Gardiner, 1996). Similarly social services may incur costs through having to become involved with a child directly, or indirectly, following exclusion, whether or not the child enters public care (see also chapter 5).

Cohen and Hughes (1994) have demonstrated the impact of exclusion within the excluded child's family, aggravating financial problems and increasing emotional tension. They also showed that excluded children may be placed at increased physical and emotional risk, a graphic illustration provided by Alderson (1994) reporting on the death of a ten-year-old boy, Joseph Kenny, who was sent home following exclusion from school for fighting, and was subsequently killed by his psychotic father.

Inter-agency approaches to prevention

It is clear that the prevention of unacceptable behaviour and prevention of exclusion should be a major priority, not only for schools themselves, but also for support services. In this section we outline strategies which have been successfully applied.

At the school level one of the consequences of school effectiveness research has been to increase awareness of the contribution schools themselves can make to the pursuit of good order (OFSTED, 1993b; DFE, 1994c). The establishment of a whole school behaviour policy is now considered critical to the efficient operation of schools and the creation of a welcoming environment conducive to teaching and learning. In contrast unsuccessful schools are likely to have failed to develop such a policy or, having developed one, to have failed effectively to implement it.

The central philosophy of an effective school behaviour policy emphasises individual self-respect, respect for others and will value individual differences (see, for example, DFE, 1994c). There will be few formal rules – emphasising positive rather than negative values and behaviour – whose existence can be vigorously defended and collectively owned, and a range of appropriate rewards and sanctions and withdrawal of 'privileges' for rule infringement. These principles will underwrite policies and procedures towards equal opportunities, disability, racial and sexual discrimination and bullying. The policy will also permeate the curriculum and ensure that pupils' experiences in the classroom are consistent with the school's policy. (Examples of how this can be achieved in relation to disability are given in chapter 8.) An effective school behaviour policy:

•   balances individual rights with responsibilities towards others, including respect for their property and towards the school and the wider environment;
•   promotes qualities of fairness, trust and honesty;
•   utilises language which is unambiguous and capable of being understood by all members of the school community;
•   identifies the rewards for achievement in a broad range of activities (and not merely recognition of academic excellence) and exemplary behaviour, for example, by public commendations, letters to pupils' parents or carers, display of pupils' work, presentations of certificates or other tangible awards at both individual and group level;
•   provides for a sufficiently wide range of sanctions which are applied fairly, consistently and in accordance with due process, which prevent premature use of 'heavy end' punishments such as exclusion, through the application of an inadequate tariff regime;
•   provides routine acknowledgement and valuing of pupil attendance and punctuality;
•   ensures that lessons will be properly planned, providing appropriate stimulation and challenge. Teachers will have appropriate expectations of pupils' attainment, and will encourage and respect pupil contributions and views.

The policy will also cover breaks and lunch-times and movement between lessons, which will necessarily involve ancillary staff such as secretarial and lunch-time supervisory staff and emphasise self-discipline among pupils.

Arguably the process by which a policy is developed, introduced and implemented is more important than its content. The most effective means of promoting ownership of and commitment to the policy by all members of the school community is to ensure their active involvement in all stages of its progress. Samson and Hart (1995) describe a four-stage process involving all members of the school community which characterises the development of behaviour policies in schools in Tameside: information gathering; feedback and identification of priorities; policy formulation and implementation, and evaluation. A wide variety of ways of involving different groups within the school can be utilised such as: reports; parents' newsletters; the school prospectus; the school annual report; parents', staff, school council and governors' meetings; INSET; assemblies and tutorial time. Finally, once a behavioural policy is in place and being implemented, it needs to be subject to regular review and evaluation to ensure that it is being applied consistently and fairly and that it is securing the desired objectives.

Transitional work may be undertaken to prepare primary school leavers for secondary school, in an effort to dispel the inevitable myths and fantasies about life in a larger school and the transition from being the oldest (and usually biggest) children in the school to becoming the youngest (and smallest). Former primary school pupils who have successfully transferred to secondary school, especially those in Year 7, can visit their former schools and talk to Year 6 pupils about their experiences of their first year in the secondary school. Schools can arrange for this to continue into the new school year to ensure a successful transition for new pupils and to encourage a sense of responsibility and consideration of others in older pupils.

Similar practices may be employed in a more targeted way. Older pupils may support and act as mentors to particular younger or disadvantaged pupils, for example, those with 'special educational needs' and other disabilities, those who may be prone to bullying and those whose past attendance or behaviour in primary school may give cause for concern. The high correlation between disaffection, poor behaviour and high levels of exclusion and low levels of academic attainment, especially literacy, are now well documented. In the longer term the task of ensuring adequate literacy skills rests squarely with primary schools. In the meantime, however, there are many children in secondary schools who lack the basic skills necessary to tackle the curriculum with any degree of confidence or likelihood of success. Those secondary schools which have eschewed the undoubted benefit of selecting their pupils according to academic attainment need, as a matter of urgency, to take remedial preventive action to improve the literacy competence of their least successful pupils through all available means, for example, paired reading and structured reading involving 'special educational needs' staff, classroom assistants, older pupils, volunteers and parents. They should also modify the curriculum where necessary for individual pupils to meet specific learning needs.

At the point at which disruption has occurred, the school's procedures need to ensure that difficult situations do not escalate through inappropriate responses. All teachers should be equipped, through INSET, to diffuse, rather than aggravate, tension. In the most serious instances of physical violence and sexual assault the pupil's immediate removal from the school will be the most appropriate course of action, although such circumstances should be extremely rare. Some schools have found it useful to provide opportunity for 'time out' either with a senior member of staff or in a part of the school specifically set aside for the purpose and under staff supervision. Some schools have also successfully introduced in-school units offering a short structured programme aimed at ensuring the pupil's return to the classroom within a specified period of time.

Some schools have also developed arrangements for government especially parent governors – to meet individual pupils and parents over issues of unacceptable behaviour and to discuss constructive ways forward without recourse to exclusion.

Bourgault (1991) describes an alternative to pupil exclusion originally developed in an American high school and successfully trialled in a number of Australian high schools. The 'parent shadowing' scheme involves the parent of a pupil whose behaviour would otherwise have resulted in exclusion sitting in class with the pupil for a day. Bourgault claims that a key factor in the scheme's success is the embarrassment experienced by pupils as a result of their parent's presence in school, supporting O'Keeffe's (1994) view of the importance of parental responses in managing children's behaviour. Bourgault recognises the limitations of this type of approach. In particular parents need to be supportive of the school's efforts and have the time to spend in school. (Although his report is silent on the subject we suspect that more mothers than fathers took part in the scheme). Initial problems such as unsettling other pupils in the class and teachers' apprehensions of being under the parental spotlight appeared to be short-lived. Indeed, an additional positive outcome was the high regard participating parents had for their children's teachers. Bourgault comments on the potential flexibility of parent shadowing, for example, targeting lessons where the child's behaviour is particularly problematic rather than all lessons, and during breaks and lunchtimes. Despite its potential, parent shadowing does not appear to be an extensively used strategy, although there has been one reported successful use of a similar arrangement at Hattersley High School in Tameside (*The Times*, 1996).

The next example we provide is an exercise in mapping pupil behaviour which we initially undertook in an inner-city high school which had introduced a formalised system for recording disciplinary incidents. We analysed the referral forms issued by staff for each incident over a period of one school term and describe the project in more detail in Blyth and Milner (1996a). The information collected on the referral forms enabled us to consider factors other than the individual pupil and their behaviour and highlighted certain patterns on which senior management in the school was able to act. This sort of analysis also meant that it was possible to 'track' pupils during the school day and investigate the possibility that problems at a given point in time might have more to do with what had happened to the pupil prior to the lesson in which, or the teacher with whom, the identified problem occurred. Interestingly we found that a small number of teachers (eleven) were responsible for issuing 60 per cent of all pupil referral forms.

The finding which had most relevance for staff was the obvious connection between various vulnerabilities in the school system; a combination of an inexperienced teacher and a 'difficult' year group in the late afternoon was a recipe for disruption. The school set in motion plans to deal with this immediately, including changes to the timetable and practical support for vulnerable members of staff. The analysis also made it much easier for the school to allocate scarce resources: for example, vulnerable pupils needing individual programmes and teachers most in need of confrontation training were identified. The difference in perceptions about disruptive behaviour led to senior staff being clearer about the 'build-up' of behaviour and its consequences for pupils in order to avoid pupils viewing disciplinary events as unfair responses to what they saw as single, and often trivial, incidents. A mapping exercise such as this can be undertaken at relatively little cost since most secondary schools have necessary computer equipment for data input and analysis. We recommend it as a valuable investment of resources as it can enable a school to examine its own practices in a way which has relevance and meaning for all staff; which helps the school to develop its own strategies rather than have them handed down from 'on high'; and to decide how its own resources can best be used.

So far we have discussed initiatives which are essentially in-school ones, although to be successful these clearly need to involve the cooperation of all members of the school community itself and external support staff. There are, in addition, contributions which external support agencies can make, although this contribution is not always recognised by schools at all and, when it is, support is sometimes not sought sufficiently early, and on occasions the support requested is not forthcoming (OFSTED, 1996b). Similarly, Parsons *et al.* (1994) observe that inter-agency cooperation to support an excluded pupil is poor before, during and after the exclusion. The evidence indicates, therefore, that much more attention needs to be paid to developing effective mediation not only between school and family but also between agencies within the welfare network.

CHAPTER 10

Protecting children from abuse and exploitation

Introduction

Teachers are the recipients of many mixed messages about their role in relation to children and the value of their work. They are the main workers in the 'business' of education, which is expected to be run cheaply and efficiently, yet they are to 'produce' educated and well socialised children. At the same time as their 'business' is trimmed down in terms of support services, their pastoral role has become more formalised. In a high court judgement delivered as a consequence of industrial action taken by teachers, Mr Justice Scott stated: 'The professional obligations of teachers are not confined to the imparting of academic knowledge to the pupils. The relationship between a teacher and his or her pupils goes further. There are obligations of discipline and care . . . to fail [to perform these duties] would not simply be a breach of common humanity, but would also be a breach of the professional obligations of the teacher' (Sim v Rotherham Metropolitan BC and other actions (1986), p. 405).

Following the court's decision the government imposed specific duties on teachers as part of a new employment contract (Education (School Teachers' Pay and Conditions of Employment) Order 1987). This order included: promoting the well-being of children; communicating and cooperating with persons and bodies outside the school; and, safeguarding children's health and safety. Up to this point teachers had viewed their role in child protection as largely one of detection and referral to specialist services (see, for example, AMMA, 1987; Maher, 1987) but the specific duties in the Order paved the way for the more extensive roles and duties school staff were to be allocated.

The mandate to protect

The mandate to prevent, detect and manage child abuse operates at international, national and community levels. For example, Article 19 of the UN Convention on the Rights of the Child states: 'such protective measures should, as appropriate, include effective procedures for the establishment of social programmes to provide the necessary support for the child and *those who have the care of the child*' (our emphasis).

At a national level the Children Act 1989 establishes the

paramountcy of the welfare of the child as a primary principle and the role of school staff was laid down in government guidance, such as *Working Together* (Home Office *et al.*, 1991), identifying specific tasks for teachers and school nurses and providing the context for joint working with social services' social workers. Local procedural guidelines, while varying slightly between different administrative areas, identify each school's responsibility for designating a member of staff to liaise with social services and attend case conferences and other meetings, as well as prescriptions to help prevent abuse via the PSE curriculum and safety teaching.

Despite appearing to create even more extra work for teachers already experiencing increased workloads, this represents a formalisation of existing procedures rather than a change in the task itself. Caring and teaching have never been activities which could easily be separated: 'During my years as a teacher and head teacher in nursery and primary schools, I was aware that child protection work was an essential part of my role, because what was happening to children outside school affected their ability to learn and to enjoy the opportunities offered to them' (David, 1993, p. 5).

Children spend a significant amount of time in schools, placing teachers and other staff in an advantageous position to detect, prevent and manage child abuse (see, for example, DHSS, 1968; London Borough of Brent, 1985; Milner and Blyth, 1988; David, 1993).

The opportunities for locating the distress of children in the school setting are both wide-ranging and unique. For example, school nurses undertake regular monitoring of children's height and weight; teachers have opportunities denied other professionals to observe children undressed during PE or swimming, and to notice the child who appears neglected, who is withdrawn, who can't concentrate on lessons because of tiredness, who exhibits behavioural disturbance, or who seems reluctant to go home at the end of the school day. Playground and lunchtime supervisors are well placed to spot the child who appears ravenously hungry or who cowers in the playground. In addition, teachers have well-developed skills in talking with children. The combination of opportunity, skills and a good relationship with a pupil increase the likelihood of teachers being the recipients of disclosures either directly or indirectly. On the other hand schools do not provide the optimum environment for teachers to listen to children who want to talk about their abusive experiences. They often lack sufficient privacy for quiet conversation, uninterrupted by other pupils or staff, and the constraints of the time-table provide few opportunities for teachers to be available to individual pupils when they are most needed.

Abuse in schools

Before we explore in more detail the role of education staff in the protection of children, we need to consider their potential contribution to child abuse and exploitation.

Taking a broad definition of child abuse, it is obvious from the number of phone calls children make to 'Childline' that schools contain teachers who are in favour of smacking (and occasionally do hit children) and who humiliate their pupils. Schools also contain pupils who behave similarly and who may not be supervised in the playground where they have opportunities to attack, humiliate or threaten other children.

Taking a narrower definition of child abuse, as outlined in *Working Together* (Home Office *et al.*, 1991) for example, schools also contain teachers who abuse children. Sometime this consists of institutional cruelty. For example, we know of a young child who was held on a leash by a playground supervisor at break times in an effort to control his 'disruptive' behaviour (the child's parents having unwillingly acceded to this as the 'only alternative' to exclusion from school). Sometimes the abuse may consist of persistent emotional ill-treatment of an unpopular pupil, or sexual abuse (e.g. Cornwall County Council, 1987). Paedophiles are known to seek employment, including teaching positions, which gives them access to vulnerable children. Although most mainstream schools may seem to offer few such opportunities to paedophiles, junior schools, where close relationships between teachers and pupils are the norm, have the potential to be dangerous places for children. Men's fears of being accused of abuse by children have resulted in many male teachers avoiding primary school posts (Charter, 1996).

Assumptions that abuse of children was only something which happened between adults and children have had to be revised in the light of research showing that a large proportion of abusers are themselves children. A community-based study of sexually abused children showed that 27 per cent of perpetrators were aged between thirteen and seventeen, with 1 per cent being aged twelve years or younger (Kelly *et al.*, 1991), while a clinical study found 36 per cent of cases involved an adolescent abuser with 20.5 per cent of cases involving an abuser aged sixteen or younger (Northern Ireland Research Team, 1991). These adolescent boys may not actually abuse in school (over two thirds of sixteen-year-old offenders' victims were under twelve years of age) and, as they lack adult abusers' skills in targeting victims, they tend to know or be related to their victims (Ryan and Lane, 1991) and, are particularly heavily represented in abuse committed by baby-sitters (Margolin, 1993). However, they will exhibit other undesirable behaviours, being characterised by social skills deficits, difficulties in anger control, withdrawn behaviour, low achievement, a history of disruption or truancy and learning difficulties, although as a group they have been found to be less delinquent than non sex offenders (for an excellent overview, see O'Callaghan and Print, 1994).

The problem of bullying in schools has received a good deal of attention on the part of schools developing their positive behaviour policies, but bullying has been used as meaning almost any distressing experience for children in school, from racism or sexist abuse to physical or sexual assault. In terms of child protection, it is possible to identify cases which require a referral to child protection services. Persistent bullies can be identified very early in school (Manning *et al.*, 1978; Peters *et al.*, 1992; Tattum, 1993) and they have a poor prognosis for violence in later life (Olweus, 1993). Although much serious bullying takes place outside the classroom, it remains the responsibility of schools with the playground being twice as likely a site than the journey to and from school (Whitney and Smith, 1993).

We should also note the risks to children of the failure to notice the distress of children who are 'in need' as well as being 'at risk', for example, teachers who fail to realise that the reason a child is unable to concentrate in class or who doesn't have homework completed or gym kit may well come from a home which fails to provide basic standards of care. Although more credence is given to children's accounts than in the past, there is the danger that 'indirect' disclosures may still be missed. For example, Milner and Blyth (1988) cite the case of 'Amanda', featured in the BBC television programme which launched 'Childline'. Pupils in 'Amanda's' class had been told to write an essay about an 'unusual lodger'. Amanda wrote about the real-life lodger in the family home who had begun to abuse her sexually. When she later returned the essay the teacher said to Amanda: 'That's disgusting. I don't want you ever to write anything like that again.'

Identifying abused and exploited children

In an attempt to help teachers identify abused pupils accurately, many books on child abuse and schools provide long lists of 'symptoms' which clinical research has shown result from abuse (see, for example, Mayes *et al.*, 1992). Unfortunately such lists are as likely to confuse as to enlighten. First, they are so exhaustive that they will include practically all pupils at some time, the 'symptoms' really adding up to nothing more than the usual indicators of pupil distress from whatever cause. Second, the 'symptoms' of abuse are not really that well understood. There are no common sets of responses. The ways in which children are affected depend on their adaptational responses and they often express different emotions simultaneously (see, for example, Jaffe *et al.*, 1990; Kelly *et al.*, 1993; Taylor *et al.*, 1993).

Neither are abused children a clearly identifiable group distinguishable from other children, although some pupil groups are particularly vulnerable, for example, disabled pupils. Historically, disabled children have been neglected in child abuse research and literature. Kennedy (1995) suggests that this is largely the result of an assumption that disabled children are less exposed to the risks of abuse than their non-disabled peers, an assumption itself based on a myth that disabled children are less likely to be targeted – either because they are not considered sufficiently physically attractive or because they are seen as objects of pity. A second myth is that, even if they are abused, the abuse is 'less harmful' to a disabled child because they do not understand or cannot feel what is happening. More insidiously, sexual abuse may be justified on the grounds that it is really an expression of affection and is likely to be the child's only experience of sexual 'pleasure' and 'gratification'. Another myth, based on the notion of the essential goodness of carers and that looking after disabled children is more demanding than the care of non-disabled children is that such people could not harm the children in their care (see chapter 8). If an allegation of intentional abuse is acknowledged, physical abuse is more likely to be explained as arising from the frustration and demands of caring for a disabled child. What is also likely is that the allegation will be disregarded on the grounds that the child is confused or their story cannot be relied upon. The credence of individuals with severe learning difficulties, who even as adults are frequently regarded as 'perpetual children', is especially vulnerable.

Despite the dearth of research on abuse and disabled children, especially that which takes account of the personal experiences of disabled people themselves (for an overview see Kelly, 1992) there is emerging evidence of two possible associations: that abuse can itself be a cause of subsequent disability and that, far from being at reduced risk of abuse compared to their non-disabled peers, disabled children face increased exposure to it. Partly this is to do with assumptions about disabled people generally (reviewed in chapter 8) which essentially see them as less than human and relatively powerless. Accordingly the inhibitions – psychological, social, moral and legal – which normally prevent the ill-treatment and exploitation of one person by another are weakened when one of them is disabled. Another factor which may increase disabled children's exposure to abuse is their increased likelihood of spending periods in institutional care of one sort or another. For example, Westcott and Cross (1996) cite the experiences of neglect and emotional abuse recounted by disabled adults who were formerly pupils in the same residential school. Westcott and Clément (1992) provide details of a 'snapshot' study of NSPCC records of abuse in residential care and educational settings over a one-year period. Of 31 children with learning and/or physical disabilities (the vast majority having learning difficulties) 21 (68 per cent) had been abused in schools. Disabled children's physical dependence and need for personal care place them in more intimate situations with adults and the routinisation of these encounters may eventually desensitise carers to the child's emotional needs or reduce inhibitions which protect against physical abuse and sexual exploitation (Westcott, 1993; Morris, 1995). Disabled children are also more likely to be cared for by a larger number of carers, thus providing wider opportunities for potential abusers.

Disabled children's powerlessness, dependency and inability to take evasive action, call for help, or even see their abuser if they have a visual impairment, and the privacy of the locations in which intimate interactions with carers usually take place (e.g. toilets, bathrooms or bedrooms) provide many opportunities for abuse to take place. The chances of detection are also reduced where learning and communication difficulties mean that the child is either unlikely to be able to tell anyone else what has happened or their efforts to do so go unheard or are misinterpreted. Kennedy (1995) notes that child protection workers are likely to adopt one of two, equally unhelpful, perceptions of disabled children. Either they will adopt the 'children first' principle which sees disabled children as indistinguishable from non-disabled children and apply inappropriate and inadequate interview methods and techniques, or they will see disabled children as distinctly different, people with whom they are insufficiently equipped to communicate.

An issue which has not generally been recognised as a child protection one, but which we consider should be, concerns the employment of children. Research by Lavalette *et al.* (1995) has shown that up to half of all fourteen and fifteen year olds are employed at any one time, and nearly three quarters have had jobs at some time. While in principle school-age children in employment are protected by national legislation (the Children and Young Persons Act 1933) and local by-laws which limit the number of hours a child may work; and specify the minimum age at which a child may work, starting and finishing times, and the nature of work which young people may perform, Lavalette *et al.* (1995) have demonstrated that the vast majority of these young people are being employed illegally. Over 90 per cent do not have the LEA work permit required by law (which ensures at least some oversight of the nature of work being done and the conditions under which it is being done); over one third work before 7 a.m. and between 40 and 63 per cent after 7 p.m. (the earliest and latest legal times for children to be working during school time), and up to 20 per cent of children under the age of thirteen (the legal minimum age at which children can be employed) have a job. The impact of employment on children's health and education and their exposure to accidents are poorly documented in Britain, although American research (Greenberger and Steinberg, 1986) has shown both its advantages (providing valuable learning experiences, introducing children to the adult world of work and relationships, and encouraging them to develop autonomy and responsibility) and disadvantages (exposure to accidents and tiredness associated with working excessive hours). Other British research (Pond and Searle, 1991) also noted that many school-age children were working to alleviate family poverty. Despite the fact that the primary legislation is over sixty years old, the government has not regarded the employment of school children as problematic. The more stringent Employment of Children Act 1973 was never implemented and, as recently as 1994 (HMSO, 1994), the government indicated that it saw no need to amend existing arrangements. However, it has been obliged to do so following the issue of a Directive from the Council of the European Union (1994) (DOH, 1995c) and, in March 1997, new regulations (the Health and Safety (Young Persons) Regulations 1997) came into force, providing a greater emphasis on the assessment of risk to young people engaged in both remunerative employment and work experience placements.

Arguably greater protection from exploitation of children in employment will come from greater vigilance on the part of those who are in regular contact with children and by more effective enforcement of legislation, although the latter is not helped by the fragmented responsibility for enforcing the legislation between LEAs (usually the education welfare service acting on the LEA's behalf), the police, local authority environmental health services and the Health and Safety Executive, and the government's reluctance to acknowledge the resource implications of LEAs affording greater priority to monitoring and enforcement.

Domestic violence and child abuse

Increasingly, the links between domestic violence and child abuse are becoming clearer although the way in which violence is transmitted intergenerationally is not a simple matter of violent, 'multi-problem' families providing a cycle of violence in which boys learn to become aggressors and girls victims, although there is some truth in this with regard to boys. Morley and Mullender (1994) review the research, concluding that:

- where there is physical child abuse, the likelihood is very high that the mother is also being physically abused;
- where there is domestic violence, the child abuse is much more likely to be physical;
- where there is domestic violence, the father is typically also the child's abuser;
- abused mothers of abused children do not usually come from disorganised or violent families of origin;
- mothers who are the victims of domestic violence are more likely to have their children removed;
- professionals fail to acknowledge the existence of domestic violence at the same time as they blame women for the abuse of their children.

The common experiences of children subject to domestic violence and child abuse are male domination and female subordination (Kelly, 1994). Schools may reflect these processes of domination and subordination without providing any scope for challenging them. It needs to be remembered that domestic violence knows no class boundaries so any school is likely to contain not only pupils who are experiencing domestic violence but also staff who are either offenders or victims.

Any school hoping to tackle child abuse needs, therefore, to recognise its own potential for contributing to the problem. It is not simply a case of the occasional paedophile preying on vulnerable pupils, but of opportunities for abusive adults to use the organisation of the school as a vehicle for the expression of their violence. For example, the Cornwall primary school head teacher convicted of numerous sexual offences against pupils over a ten-year period adopted a dominating style of authority over staff as well as pupils which left his staff disunited and powerless to take action (Cornwall County Council, 1987). Therefore, schools are unlikely to be able to take effective action to protect children unless they are first able to establish a non-abusive organisation. Without this, a school's child protection system could only lead to secondary (institutional) abuse.

Women protection and child protection

Kelly (1994) argues that 'women protection' is frequently the most effective form of child protection so the first action a school needs to take is to examine how it treats all its female staff. Although there have been few studies on female staff in schools generally, we do know that they are subordinated in many ways. For example, female lunchtime supervisors had to take court action to bring their pay into line with that of male caretakers, and there is a great deal of evidence of the ways in which female teachers are disadvantaged in all areas of school life. The problem is that masculinity is defined negatively – on the basis of what it is not, that is, femininity (Brannon and David, 1976; Segal, 1990) – and this means that male teachers need to reduce the power of female teachers to maintain their own masculinities in much the same way as male pupils needs female pupils in the class to boost their motivation to achieve academically.

This manifests itself as female teachers experiencing different discipline problems with male pupils to male teachers (see, for example, Marshall, 1996) and being undermined or 'rescued' by male teachers. For example: 'I find myself being undermined by male colleagues – sometimes they think they are "protecting" me. For example, there's a teacher in the room across from me. Whenever the noise level in my lessons reaches a certain point, he'll burst into the room to quieten down the class or tell them off. It makes me feel totally stripped of authority in front of the boys' (female teacher cited in Askew and Ross, 1988, p. 60).

Additionally, male teachers find it difficult to tolerate the assertiveness of male pupils, particularly where this is directed at female teachers in public areas of the school and particularly where the pupils are adolescent African-Caribbean boys. While they often 'protect' female teachers from what they perceive as sexual harassment, they rarely make the same efforts to protect female pupils from the 'slag' culture of the boys' definitions of femininity in school (see, for example, Lees, 1986; Haywood and Mac an Ghaill, 1996) and anti-bullying packs pay no attention to sexism as part of institutionalised bullying. For example, the DFE pack (1994g) explicitly includes race and ethnicity as components of bullying but ignores sexism.

Where women are consistently demeaned in schools it is difficult to devise a child protection system which will be convincing for the victims of abuse. Why should they disclose to a teacher who is seen as powerless in the face of male oppression? A discipline mapping exercise as suggested in chapter 9 would aid the establishment of a whole school approach to child protection in which female staff could become useful role models, as is developing in the youth service (e.g. Hainsworth, 1996).

Women provide more effective role models for boys on the grounds that 'the lads' problems were not that they were starved of male role models, it was that they were saturated with them' (Campbell, 1993, p. 323). David offers some useful advice on how a whole school approach to child protection can develop a 'listening approach' with shared decision making and supportive networks (David, 1993, pp. 87–9) and whole school training exercises can be found in Milner and Blyth (1988, pp. 41–50).

Contributing to an inter-agency strategy

Having established a non-abusive child protection ethos in schools, the process following the detection of serious abuse consists of: responding to the child's distress appropriately; making notes about the incident; reporting it to a senior or designated teacher; informing the parents and support staff; referring to an appropriate social work agency; and (possibly) attending case conferences and reviews and participating in core groups (Sage, 1993; DFEE, 1995a). There are, however, potential problems at each of these stages.

- Responding to the child appropriately. As noted earlier, it is not necessarily the class teacher who is the first to detect a serious incident of abuse. For example, often a sexually abused child will tell a friend who then passes on the information to a teacher who that pupil trusts, or a member of ancillary staff notices a child wolfing food at lunchtime or sobbing in the playground. The teacher is then usually faced with talking to the pupil from the standpoint of 'I have been told . . .' and at a time when there is a lesson to be conducted. School staff, therefore, need space, time and opportunities for planning if they are to deal sensitively with these situations. Doyle (1995) offers helpful strategies for people who come across child abuse only occasionally and who need assistance in providing positive help.

- Recording. It is vital that comprehensive notes are taken at the time of the initial referral within school – child death inquiries are full of accounts of decisions being made on the basis of what later turns out to be inaccurate information (see, for example, Reder *et al.*, 1993). Early recording will mitigate the inevitable 'Chinese whisper' effect as information is passed from lunchtime supervisor to teacher to senior or designated teacher to social services. The Department for Education and Employment cautions teachers to ensure any reports distinguish between 'fact, observation, allegation and opinion' (DFEE, 1995a, p. 8). It is also good practice at this stage to take out the pupil's file and begin to make notes for a more formal report. The DFEE advises that reports should 'focus on the child's educational progress and achievements, attendance, behaviour, participation, relations with other children and, where appropriate, the child's appearance. If relevant, reports should include what is known about the child's relations with his or her family and the family structure' (DFEE, 1995a, p. 8). In addition we would suggest that such reports could also usefully contain information about any health concerns, details about family contact with the school and whether there are any siblings who may also be at risk, together with any comments or observations provided by colleagues.

• Reporting to a senior or designated teacher. At this stage, the responsible member of staff can usefully convene a meeting, including relevant school and support staff, to gather as much information as possible before making an official referral. Few cases are so urgent that action needs to be immediate, although education welfare officers and child protection workers will know that a surprising number of concerns are first raised late on a Friday afternoon or on the last day before a school holiday! Time to reflect at this stage not only aids the preparation of a full and accurate report and identification of key staff for subsequent management stages but will also detect those increasingly common referrals which have more to do with short-cutting the statementing process rather than child abuse (Milner, 1993). This stage also represents the beginning of good intra-agency cooperation and planning.

• Informing parents. It is usually left to the investigating social worker to inform parents, although on almost any other occasion the school would take responsibility to contact parents. Indeed, schools are best placed to do so as they may have a relationship with parents and their records will also contain information about which parent can be contacted during the school day. In passing this responsibility to social workers they avoid two major problems for themselves but worsen them for others. First, is the ill defined legal status of the investigative social worker's right to examine the child. Although the Kimberley Carlile inquiry (London Borough of Greenwich, 1987) criticised the senior social worker, Martin Ruddock, for not having a clearly under-nourished child examined for possible injury, and made recommendations about the examination of children, the Children Act 1989 did little to make this easier. Without parental permission, the social worker must apply to a court for a child assessment order, a process which takes time and may leave the child in danger or precipitously raise the stakes. School teachers, by virtue of their responsibility to care for pupils, have parental rights which they could exercise at this stage.

Second, informing parents is fraught with potential difficulties. Most local authority procedures reflect these, stating that parents must be informed before a child is examined except in cases of sexual abuse. But the main problem here is that alleged abusers are unlikely to respond to requests that their children are medically examined because of suspected abuse. Such parents usually respond angrily, and not infrequently with threats of violence. Some parents have already made their potential violence known to schools earlier; for example, Kimberley Carlile's step-father, Nigel Hall, had made a point of intimidating all the professionals, including the school teacher (London Borough of Greenwich, 1987). As recent tragedies of violence in schools perpetrated by unwelcome visitors have shown, one of the most pressing issues is how to deal with confrontations with possibly violent men so that schools can provide a safe environment. This is a matter of some urgency not only for worker protection but also for child and mother protection and to avoid the tendency to home in on the 'softer' target of the mother (DOH, 1995d; Milner, 1996).

• Referring to social services. In most instances this consists of a telephone call to the duty social worker and the relief of handing the problem over to someone else. However, the multi-agency strategy means that plans will need to be made about subsequent case conference attendance, deciding who will attend and timetabling for this, and preparing reports. Preparation at this stage can save much time later.

• Case conferences. As child death inquiries have consistently identified inadequate information flow as a factor in the poor management of child abuse cases, decision making in the case conference has become central, with inter-agency cooperation being seen as the way decision making can be more properly focused and objective. However, there are problems with depending on a group to make better quality decisions than individuals. For example, inter-agency cooperation is problematic (for an overview see Blyth and Milner, 1990; Hallett and Birchall, 1992). A particular problem for schools is that where there is a designated teacher who attends case conferences, they will soon become part of a group of 'professional acquaintances' who attend conferences regularly, tending to the risk of collusion.

Even more serious is the problem of increasing evidence, challenging accepted wisdom, that two heads are *not* better than one. Extensive psychological research shows that groups make more extreme decisions than individuals in the direction of either risky or cautious decision making (for an overview, see Davis *et al.*, 1992). This is particularly so when the group is faced with a choice between unattractive alternatives, such as is usual in child protection where the decision is between leaving the child at home with parents (a decision which is desirable but carries a higher risk of abuse) or taking the child into care (a decision which is undesirable but which carries a lower risk of abuse). The tendency to avoid the certain loss involved in the first choice is exaggerated by group processes which are stronger in groups which have to reach consensus and are collusive – factors which are highly likely in case conferences (for an overview, see Kelly and Milner, 1996). This means that case conference participants tend to lose sight of the possible losses to the child in their efforts to keep a family together and teachers find that they are pressurised into accepting group reassurances about the child's safety which they do not share; that their information is disregarded when it does not fit with the group's preferences; and sometimes they are not invited to subsequent meetings.

As inter-agency cooperation in itself offers no intrinsic safeguards for children's safety or welfare teachers need to feel confident in their unique contribution to the inter-agency strategy. They can best prepare for this by bringing to the case conference the detailed written report. Schools may well have information which no other individual or agency possesses. Teachers are not only one of the few professional groups in direct and regular contact with abused children, but also – like health visitors and school nurses – are in routine contact with the much larger group of non-abused and non-disadvantaged children, and can, therefore, provide a perspective based on day-to-day exposure to a more representative cross-section of children than that experienced by most social workers and child protection specialists. Teachers are also in a good position to represent the view of the child and know what the school can offer the child in the wake of abuse. Moving the child, giving them a 'fresh start', may not be the best option when the loss of the stability and social support which can be provided by the school is taken into account. Even if the child needs to be removed from home and placed in a residential or foster home further away from the school, the teacher can challenge the assumption that a change of placement should inevitably result in a change of school (see also chapter 5). Teachers should also insist that they are members of the core group which will manage the child protection plan.

• Core groups. As teachers have responsibility for many children, they can make a good case that core group meetings are held at a time and place convenient for them. Core group decisions need to be monitored carefully as there is evidence that they often persist with a care plan even when one vital component goes missing, usually the cooperation of the abuser (Hallett and Birchall, 1992). Where this happens, the issue should be taken back to the full case conference. Where a child is admitted to the care system, child protection issues remain for the teacher who may well be the only person who retains a strong interest in the child's education. As we have shown in chapter 5, the research literature on the education of children in the care system makes depressing reading.

Despite initial enthusiasm about the Children Act 1989, child protection issues have priority over children 'in need' and probably the teacher's most effective work will take place in the area of prevention.

Preventing abuse

In practice the school's role in preventing abuse has tended to consist mainly of safety teaching, especially in primary schools, which it has been relatively easy to 'add on' to existing teaching on road safety, 'stranger danger' and how to cope with emergencies such as fire, accidents and getting lost. Much of this safety teaching was influenced by the pioneering work of Elliott (1985, 1987) which sought to protect children from sexual abuse by explaining to them that they have rights and introducing them to distinctions between 'good' and 'bad' touches and secrets. The emphasis here was on making children safe by teaching them to say 'no'. There have been no parallel programmes aimed at preventing other forms of abuse. Although anti-bullying programmes (e.g. the anti-bullying pack, *Bullying: Don't Suffer in Silence* (DFE, 1994g)) go some way towards preventing the physical abuse of children by other children, while still emphasising speaking out, there are limits to the effectiveness of this approach. For example, teaching a child to 'say no' to neglect is unlikely to be productive. Mainstream safety and preventive education programmes focusing on strategies which depend on the child's ability to call for assistance, take evasive action or physically escape are of limited value to the disabled child with motor or sensory impairments. David (1993) comments that expecting children to protect themselves against the unwanted attacks or assaults of a bigger child or adult is unreasonable. It also focuses attention on the responsibilities of victims rather than offenders; we have found numerous examples of primary school age pupils being prescribed safety training by case conference care plans as an alternative to removing the perpetrator from the home. If social services and schools cannot deal effectively with the resistances of violent men, how can children be expected to do so?

And safety training assumes that 'go and tell' and 'say no' are the preferred ways of dealing with safety issues when, in fact, children use multiple strategies for dealing with abuse. Kelly *et al.* (1993) found that sexually abused children were more likely to tell their mother and peers than teachers and that this was a strategy more frequently used by girls.

Boys were more likely to try to get away from the abuse. The children also used a variety of resistance strategies including telling, crying, physical resistance, running away, avoidance, screaming/making a noise, and threatening to tell. Kelly *et al.* (1993) argue that safety trainers need to recognise the range of strategies that are used, enable peers to respond appropriately when told, help children identify which adults they could ask for help and how threatening to tell can be most effectively used as a resistance strategy.

As well as taking a more sophisticated approach to safety training and increasing peer support systems in school, school staff can increase their credibility as people who will not only listen but also actively help. The major issue here is the need to avoid the subordination of women discussed earlier but there are also some simple practical measures which can be adopted which will demonstrate to pupils that the whole school is a safe environment (see chapters 8 and 9 for further discussion of these issues).

Within the curriculum there are a number of ways in which PSE can be extended to prevent child abuse. For example, Mardon (1996) describes a parenting course for young fathers looking at both the practical and emotional aspects of child care provided in a young offenders' institute. She argues that many of the young men are intending to bring up their children in ways that are qualitatively different from the ways in which they were brought up, but that their lack of education and poor social and life skills made this a problem for them. As one young man commented: 'I had a terrible relationship with my father and even now I don't ever want to see him again. I don't want my baby to feel like that about me. The course helps you to handle things like that. . . . It really gives you the view that you should share the responsibility of bringing up your child' (Mardon, 1996, pp. 139–40). These young men have a desire to be different, but it is not necessary to wait until they become convicted offenders before providing them with parenting courses. Mardon says that the suggestion that boys are not interested in parenting courses is contradicted by the piloting of a short course for young men who were not already fathers which was well received. She believes that the single-sex group setting of the institution is essential to prevent the young men appearing 'soft' when they discuss their feelings. Elsewhere we have outlined the role of schools in teaching for 'responsible manhood' (Milner and Blyth, 1988).

Violence can be prevented before it happens by altering attitudes, values and behaviours. Some schools are attempting this by involving Women's Aid groups on planning anti-violence work, particularly in conjunction with work on bullying and racism (Higgins, 1994), while a more advanced preventive programme has been developed in Canada (for an overview see Mullender, 1994). In elementary schools a key idea is to base activities around a violence awareness and prevention week involving all school and community personnel. The whole curriculum for this age group covers learning about different forms of violence and their effects, personal safety planning, expressing feelings, assertiveness and self-worth while respecting others – this latter element being often missing from British safety programmes.

Work in secondary school has an additional emphasis on pupils' own relationships, many of which are already violent. Pupils themselves are fully involved with a pupil planning committee for the programme as a whole and specific schemes for pupils to offer mediation and peer counselling. One imaginative idea is for a positively rather than a negatively oriented sanction to apply when a pupil breaks the non-violence code. For example, rather than being excluded, the pupil receives an in-school suspension in which they are required to attend sessions on conflict resolution or interpersonal skills. The training pack emphasises that anti-violence work can be integrated into the curriculum from history to maths (Sudermann *et al.*, 1994).

The main drawback with the pack is that racism and homophobia are not given sufficient prominence (Mullender, 1994) and rather more emphasis is given to pupil–pupil and pupil–family abuse than to teacher–pupil abuse. It is nonetheless a comprehensive pack which offers a whole school–community programme, and if used in Britain would provide a way of involving all members of the school and support networks, and not limit the responsibility of schools to that of teachers alone.

Kennedy provides examples of the use of appropriate communications techniques with abused disabled children (e.g. Kennedy and Gordon, 1993; Marchant and Page, 1993), and argues that effective preventive programmes must recognise disabled children's potential vulnerability to abuse and emphasise their empowerment. These ideas are reinforced by Middleton (1996) and Westcott and Cross (1996) who further propose increased cooperation and exchange of knowledge and expertise between child care and disability 'specialists' as a means of ensuring that the child protection system affords more effective safeguards to disabled children.

Many schools serving deprived catchment areas have additional problems where the issues around child protection have much more to do with poverty and neglect – and pupils who come to school undernourished and inadequately clothed. A referral of an impoverished, neglected child is likely to result in professionals regarding this as a matter of parental inadequacy with interventions designed to teach parents (mostly lone mothers) budgeting skills or educate them about the health risks of poor diet and smoking (Graham, 1993). These measures do little to improve pupils' abilities to cope in school and ignore the efforts of many of these schools which do their best to offset disadvantage. Additionally, there is evidence that community education for mothers in deprived areas is helpful. Flett (1993) describes an early childhood education programme in a disadvantaged community in Scotland which promoted a clear partnership between local parents and professionals which developed educational opportunities. In principle, greater school autonomy makes it easier for individual schools to set in train community education programmes which have the potential to increase the effectiveness of schools and permit the flexible use of budgets, although we recognise that education reforms have, in practice, made it more difficult for schools to budget for child protection and, together with other welfare reforms, have made coordinated inter-agency provision less easy to deliver (National Commission of Inquiry into the Prevention of Child Abuse, 1996).

Bibliography

Acker, S. (1981) 'Women and education', in Hartnett, A. (ed.) *The Social Sciences in Education*, London: Hutchinson.

Advisory Centre for Education (1992) 'Exclusions', *ACE Bulletin*, 47, pp. 4–5.

Advisory Centre for Education (1995) *Governors' Handbook*, London: Advisory Centre for Education.

Ahmad, B. (1991) *Black Perspectives on Social Work*, Birmingham: Venture Press.

Alderson, K. (1994) 'Voices drove man to kill children with hammer', *The Times*, 24 September, p. 6.

Aldridge, J. and Becker, S. (1993) *Children Who Care – Inside the World of Young Carers*, Loughborough: Loughborough University.

Aldridge, J. and Becker, S. (1994) *My Child, My Carer – the Parents' Perspective*, Loughborough: Loughborough University.

Alexander, H. (1995) *Young Carers and HIV*, Edinburgh: Children in Scotland.

Allen, T. (1994) 'The exclusion of pupils from school: the need for reform', *Journal of Social Welfare and Family Law*, 2, pp. 145–62.

Arnott, M., Raab, C. and Munn, P. (1996) 'Devolved management: variations of response in Scottish School Boards', in Pole, C. and Chawla-Duggan, R. (eds) *Reshaping Education in the 1990s: Perspectives on Secondary Schooling*, London: Falmer Press.

Arora, C. M. J. and Thompson, D. A. (1987) 'Defining the bully for a secondary school', *Educational and Child Psychology*, 4, 3, pp. 110–20.

Aronsson, K. (1991) 'Social interaction and the recycling of evidence', in Coupland, M., Giles, H. and Weimann, J. M. (eds) *'(Mis)communication' and Problematic Talk*, London: Sage.

Askew, S. and Ross, C. (1988) *Boys Don't Cry: Boys and Sexism in Education*, Milton Keynes: Open University Press.

Assistant Masters and Mistresses Association (1987) *Sexual Issues, the Law and the Teacher's Responsibility*, London: Assistant Masters and Mistresses Association.

Association of Chief Education Social Workers and National Association of Social Workers in Education (1991) *Code of Principles and Practice*.

Association of Directors of Social Services (1978) *Social Work Services for Children in Schools*, London: ADSS.

Association of Metropolitan Authorities (1995) *Reviewing Special Educational Needs: Report of the AMA Working Party on Special Educational Needs*, London: AMA.

Audit Commission (1994) *Seen But Not Heard: Co-ordinating Community Child Health and Social Services for Children in Need*, London: HMSO.

Audit Commission (1996a) *Planning and Supply of School Places and Parent Satisfaction*, London: HMSO.

Audit Commission (1996b) *Young People and Crime*, London: Audit Commission.

Audit Commission and HMI (1992) *Getting in on the Act: Provision for Pupils with Special Educational Needs*, London: HMSO.

Ball, S. (1990) *Politics and Policy-making in Education*, London: Routledge.

Ball, S. (1993) 'Education markets, choice and social class: the market as a class strategy in the UK and the USA', *British Journal of Sociology of Education*, 14, 1, pp. 3–19.

Barber, J. (1991) *Beyond Casework*, London: BASW/Macmillan.

Barkley, R. A. (1990) *Attention Deficit Hyperactivity Disorder,* New York: Guildford Press.

Barnard, H. (1969) *A History of English Education*, London: University of London Press.

Barnes, C. (1994) *Disabled People in Britain and Discrimination: A Case for Anti-Discrimination Legislation*, London: Hurst & Co.

Barstow, P., Cochrane, R. and Hur, J. (1993) *Evaluation of Conductive Education for Children with Cerebral Palsy*, Birmingham: Department for Education and University of Birmingham.

BBC (1996) *Panorama*, 4 November.

Becker, S. (1993) 'Children who care', in Carers National Association *Young Carers – Strategies and Structures: Working with Young Carers*. Conference Report, October, 1993, London: Carers National Association.

Becker, S. and Aldridge, J. (1995) 'Young carers in Great Britain', in Becker, S. (ed.) *Young Carers in Europe: An Exploratory Cross-National Study in Britain, France, Sweden and Germany*, Loughborough: Loughborough University.

Bee, H. (1985) *The Developing Person* (5th Edition), London: Harper & Row.

Bennathan, M. (1992) 'The care and education of troubled children', *Young Minds Newsletter*, 10, March, pp. 1–7.

Bentovim, A. (1991) 'Significant Harm in Context' in Adcock, M., White, R. and Hollows, A. (eds) *Significant Harm*, Croydon: Significant Publications.

Berg, I. (1996) 'Unauthorised absence from school', in Berg, I. and Nursten, J. (eds) *Unwillingly to School* (4th edn), London: Gaskell.

Berg, I., Hullin, R., McGuire, R. and Tyrer, S. (1977) 'Truancy and the courts: research note', *Journal of Child Psychology and Psychiatry*, 18, pp. 359–65.

Berg, I., Consterdine, M., Hullin, R., McGuire, R. and Tyrer, S. (1978) 'The effect of two randomly allocated court procedures on truancy', *British Journal of Criminology*, 18, 3, pp. 232–44.

Berliner, W. (1990) 'Handicapped pupils: the scandal of the lies parents are told', *The Observer*, 4 February, p. 52.

Berridge, D. (1985) *Children's Homes*, Oxford: Basil Blackwell.

Berridge, D. and Cleaver, H. (1987) *Foster Home Breakdown*, Oxford: Basil Blackwell.

Biehal, N., Clayden, J., Stein, M. and Wade, J. (1992) *Prepared for Living? A Survey of Young People Leaving the Care of Three Local Authorities*, London: National Children's Bureau.

Bilsborrow, S. (1992) *'You grow up fast as well . . .' Young Carers on Merseyside*, London: Carers National Association, Personal Social Services Society and Barnados.

Blaxter, M. (1976) *The Meaning of Disability: A Sociological Study of Impairment*, London: Heinemann.

Blyth, E. and Milner, J. (1987a) 'The juvenile court and non-attendance at school', *Justice of the Peace*, 151, 51, 19 December, pp. 854–7.

Blyth, E. and Milner, J. (1987b) 'Non-attendance and the law: the confused role of the social services and education departments', in Reid, K. (ed.) *Combating School Absenteeism*, London: Hodder & Stoughton.

Blyth, E. and Milner, J. (1988) 'Is education welfare social work?' *Practice*, 1, 4, pp. 339–54.

Blyth, E. and Milner, J. (1990) 'Interagency cooperation', in Violence Against Children Study Group, *Taking Child Abuse Seriously*, London: Unwin Hyman.

Blyth, E. and Milner, J. (1996a) 'Black boys excluded from school: race or masculinity issues?' in Blyth, E. and Milner, J. (eds) *Exclusion from School: Inter-professional Issues for Policy and Practice*, London: Routledge.

Blyth, E. and Milner, J. (1996b) 'Exclusions: trends and issues', in Blyth, E. and Milner, J. (eds) *Exclusion from School: Inter-professional Issues for Policy and Practice*, London: Routledge.

Blyth, E. and Milner, J. (1996c) 'Social work in education: towards a new agenda', *Improving Attendance, Achievement and Motivation 1995 National Conference Report,* Leeds: Leeds City Council and the University of Huddersfield.

Blyth, E. and Milner, J. (1996d) 'Unsaleable goods and the education market', in Pole, C. and Chawla-Duggan, R. (eds) *Reshaping Education in the 1990s: Perspectives on Secondary Schooling*, London: Falmer Press.

Blyth, E., Saleem, T. and Scott, M. (1995) *Kirklees Young Carers Project, October 1994–June 1995: Report to Kirklees Metropolitan Council*, Huddersfield: The University of Huddersfield.

Blyth, E., Saleem, T. and Scott, M. (1996) *Kirklees Young Carers Project, July 1995–July 1996: Report to Kirklees Metropolitan Council*, Huddersfield: The University of Huddersfield.

Botvin, G. (1995) 'Drug abuse prevention in school settings', in Botvin, G., Schinke, S. and Orlandi, M. (eds) *Drug Abuse Prevention with Multiethnic Youth*, Sage: Thousand Oaks.

Bourdieu, P. and Passeron, J. C. (1990) *Reproduction in Education, Society and Culture*, London: Sage.

Bourgault, G. (1991) 'Parent shadowing: an effective alternative sanction for some students who pose discipline problems', *Pastoral Care*, 9, 3, pp. 43–5.

Bowen, D. E. (1985) 'Education – Whose Care? A consideration of the educational effect of making care orders in respect of non-attenders at school', unpublished M.Sc. dissertation, Cranfield: Cranfield Institute of Technology.

Bowis, J. (1995) 'The Department of Health and young carers', in *Young Carers: Back Them Up*. Report of a conference organised jointly by Community Care and Carers National Association at BMA House, London, 17 November, London: Community Care and Carers National Association.

Bowlby, J. (1980) *Attachment and Loss*, Harmondsworth: Penguin.

Brandt, G. L. (1986) *The Realisation of Anti-racist Teaching*, Lewes: Falmer Press.

Brannon, R. and David, D. S. (1976) 'The male sex role: our culture's blueprint of manhood and what it's done for us lately', in David, D. S. and Brannon, R. (eds) *The Forty-Nine Per Cent Majority*, Reading, Mass: Addison-Wesley.

Bristol Child Health and Education Study (1986) 'West Indians: no link between disadvantage and attainment', *Education*, 28, p. 383.

Brown, P. (1987) *Schooling Ordinary Kids*, London: Tavistock.

Brown, S. (1996) 'Educational Change in the United Kingdom: A North–South Divide', in Pole, C. and Chawla-Duggan, R. (eds) *Reshaping Education in the 1990s: Perspectives on Secondary Schooling*, London: Falmer Press.

Bullock, R., Little, M. and Millham, S. (1993) *Going Home*, Aldershot: Dartmouth.

Bullock, R., Little, M. and Millham, S. (1994) 'Children's return from state care to school', *Oxford Review of Education*, 20, 3, pp. 307–16.

Buswell, C. (1981) 'Sexism in school routines and classroom practice', *Durham and Newcastle Research Review*, 946, pp. 195–200.

Campbell, B. (1993) *Goliath: Britain's Dangerous Places*, London: Methuen.

Carers National Association (1992) *Young Carers Link*, March.

Carers National Association (1993) *Young Carers and the Children Act 1989*, London: Carers National Association.

Carlen, P. (1987) 'Out of care, into custody: dimensions and decon-structions of the State's regulation of twenty-two young working-class women', in Carlen, P. and Worall, A. (eds) *Gender, Crime and Justice*, Milton Keynes: Open University Press.

Carlen, P., Gleeson, D. and Wardhaugh, J. (1992) *Truancy: The Politics of Compulsory Schooling*, Buckingham: Open University Press.

Carrington, B. (1986) 'Social Mobility, Ethnicity and Sport', *British Journal of Sociology*, 7, 1, pp. 3–18.

Carvel, J. and Dyer, C. (1996) 'Schools' fear as ex-pupils sue', *Guardian*, 2 December, p. 1.

Casey, B. and Smith, D. (1995) *Truancy and Youth Transitions: England and Wales Youth Cohort Study. Cohort Report No. 34*, London: Policy Studies Institute.

Central Advisory Council for Education (1963) *Half our Future* (The Newsome Report), London: HMSO.

Central Advisory Council for Education (1967) *Children and their Primary Schools* (The Plowden Report), London: HMSO.

Central Council for Education and Training in Social Work (1995) *Preventing Behaviour Problems: Practice Issues in Education Social Work: Improving Social Education and Training Nineteen*, London: CCETSW.

Channer, Y. (1995) *I am a Promise: The School Achievement of British African Caribbeans*, Stoke-on-Trent: Trentham Books.

Chapman, A. J., Smith, J. R., Foot, H. C. and Pritchard, E. (1979) 'Behavioural and sociometric indices of friendship in children', in Cook, M. and Wilson, G. (eds) *Love and Attraction*, Oxford: Pergamon.

Charter, D. (1995) 'Church school parents may lose opt-out voice', *The Times*, 28 October, p. 8.

Charter, D. (1996) 'Male teachers are shunning primary schools', *The Times*, 31 July, p. 7.

Cheung, S. Y. and Heath, A. (1994) 'After care: the education and occupation of adults who have been in care', *Oxford Review of Education*, 20, 3, pp. 361–74.

Children's Rights Development Unit (1994) *UK Agenda for Children*, London: CRDU.

Clare, J. (1993) 'The Hard Sell', *Daily Telegraph*, 12 October, p. 14.

Claxton, G. (1984) *Learn and Live*, London: Harper & Row.

Clegg, A. and Megson, B. (1976) *Children in Distress,* Harmondsworth: Penguin.

Cockburn, C. (1987) *Two-Track Training: Sex Inequalities and the Youth Training Scheme*, London: Macmillan.

Cohen, N. (1994) 'One-party Britain', *Independent on Sunday*, 3 April, p. 17.

Cohen, N. and Weir, S. (1994) 'Welcome to Quangoland', *Independent on Sunday*, 22 May, p. 9.

Cohen, R. and Hughes, M. (1994) *School's Out: The Family Perspective and School Exclusions*, London and Ilford: Family Service Units and Barnardos.

Colton, M. and Heath, A. (1994) 'Attainment and behaviour of children in care and at home', *Oxford Review of Education*, 20, 3, pp. 317–27.

Community Care and Carers National Association (1995) *Young Carers: Back Them Up*. Report of a conference organised jointly by *Community Care* and Carers National Association at BMA House,

London, 17 November, London: *Community Care* and Carers National Association.

Condon, P. (1995) cited in *The Times*, 8 July, p. 4.

Cook, A. and Campbell, B. (1981) *Sweet Freedom: the Struggle for Women's Liberation*, London: Picador.

Coombes, F. and Beer, D. (1984) *The Long Walk from the Dark*, Birmingham: National Association of Social Workers in Education.

Cooper, P., Upton, G. and Smith, C. (1991) 'Ethnic minority and gender distribution among staff and pupils with emotional and behavioural difficulties', *British Journal of Sociology of Education*, 12, pp. 77–94.

Coopers and Lybrand (1993) *Within Reach: The School Surveys*, London: NUT/Spastics Society.

Coopers and Lybrand Deloitte (1988) *Local Management of School*, *Report to the DES*, London: Coopers and Lybrand Deloitte.

Cornwall County Council (1987) *Child Abuse in Schools: Report of a Working Party on Child Abuse in Schools*, Truro: Cornwall County Council.

Council of the European Union (1994) *Council Directive 94/33/EC of 22 June 1994 on the protection of young people at work*, Brussels: Council of the European Union.

Croall, J. (1991) 'Special needs, muddled deeds', *Education Guardian*, 26 March, p. 25.

Croll, P. (1981) 'Social class, pupil achievement and classroom interaction', in Simon, B. and Willcocks, J. (eds) *Research and Practice in the Primary Classroom*, London: Routledge & Kegan Paul.

Cullen, M.-A. (1996) 'Researching Exclusions in Scotland', paper presented at 'The Prevention and Management of Exclusion from School: An Interagency Conference', University of York, 10 July, Huddersfield: Centre for Education Welfare Studies, University of Huddersfield and Society of Education Officers.

Cullingford, C. and Morrison, J. (1996) 'Who excludes whom? The personal experience of exclusion', in Blyth, E. and Milner, J. (eds) *School Exclusions: Inter-professional Issues for Policy and Practice*, London: Routledge.

Cullingford, C. and Morrison, J. (1997) 'Peer group pressure within and outside school', *British Educational Research Journal,* 23, 1, pp. 61–80.

David, T. (1993) *Child Protection and Early Years Teaching: Coping with Child Abuse*, Buckingham: Open University Press.

Davie, R., Butler, N. R. and Goldstein, H. (1972) *From Birth to Seven*, London: Longman.

Davies, L. (1984) *Pupil Power: Deviance and Gender in Schools*, Lewes: Falmer.

Davis, J. H., Kameda, T. and Stasson, M. F. (1992) 'Group risk taking: selected topics', in Yates, J. F. (ed.) *Risk-taking Behaviour*, London: Wiley.

Dearden, C. and Becker, S. (1995) *Young Carers: The Facts*, Sutton: Community Care.

Dearden, C. and Becker, S. (1996) *Young Carers at the Crossroads: An Evaluation of the Nottingham Young Carers Project*, Loughborough: Young Carers Research Group, Loughborough University.

Deem, P. (1996) 'The school, the parent, the banker and the local politician: what can we learn from the English experience of involving lay people in the site based management of schools?' in Pole, C. and Chawla-Duggan, R. (eds) *Reshaping Education in the 1990s: Perspectives on Secondary Schooling*, London: Falmer Press.

Delamont, S. (1994a) 'Sex roles and the school', in Moon, B. and Shelton Mayes, A. (eds) *Teaching and Learning in the Secondary School*, London: Routledge (in association with the Open University).

Delamont, S. (1994b) 'Sex stereotyping in the classroom', in Moon, B. and Shelton Mayes, A. (eds) *Teaching and Learning in the Secondary School*, London: Routledge (in association with the Open University).

Department for Education (1992a) *Choice and Diversity: A New Framework for Schools*. Cm 2021, London: HMSO.

Department for Education (1992b) *Education into the Next Century: The Government's Proposals for Education Explained*, London: Department for Education.

Department for Education (1992c) *Exclusions: A Discussion Paper*, London: Department for Education.

Department for Education (1993) *A New Deal for 'Out of School' Pupils*, Press Release: 126/93, London: Department for Education.

Department for Education (1994a) *Our Children's Education: The Updated Parents' Charter*, London: Department for Education.

Department for Education (1994b) *Code of Practice on the Identification and Assessment of Special Educational Needs*, London: Department for Education.

Department for Education (1994c) *Pupil Behaviour and Discipline*, Circular No. 8/94, London: Department for Education.

Department for Education (1994d) *Exclusions from School*, Circular No. 10/94, London: Department for Education.

Department for Education (1994e) *The Education by LEAs of Children Otherwise than at School*, Circular No. 11/94, London: Department for Education.

Department for Education (1994f) *School Attendance: Policy and Practice on Categorisation of Absence*, London: Department for Education.

Department for Education (1994g) *Bullying: Don't Suffer in Silence. An Anti-Bullying Pack for Schools*, London: Department for Education.

Department for Education (1995a) *GM Schools General Progress Report, Statistical Memorandum,* London: Department for Education.

Department for Education (1995b) *Statistics on School Performance Published*, DFE News, 43/95, 28 February, London: Department for Education.

Department for Education (1995c) *Grants for Education Support and Training (GEST) Scheme – Truancy and Disaffected Pupils Category: Directory of Approved Projects 1994–95*, London: Department for Education and Employment.

Department for Education and Employment (1995a) *Protecting Children from Abuse: The Role of the Education Service*, Circular 10/95. London: Department for Education and Employment.

Department for Education and Employment (1995b) *National Pupil Absence Tables 1995*, London: Department for Education.

Department for Education and Employment (1995c) *Grants for Education Support and Training (GEST) Scheme – Truancy and Disaffected Pupils Category: Directory of Approved Projects 1995–96*, London: Department for Education and Employment.

Department for Education and Employment (1996) *Grants for Education Support and Training (GEST) Programme – Truancy and Disaffected Pupils: Directory of Approved Projects 1996–97*, London: Department for Education and Employment.

Department for Education and Department of Health (1994a) *The Education of Children with Emotional and Behavioural Difficulties*, Circular No. 9/94. DH LAC (94) 9, London: Department for Education and Department of Health.

Department for Education and Department of Health (1994b) *The Education of Children Looked After by Local Authorities*, Circular No. 13/94. DH LAC (94) 11, London: Department for Education and Department of Health.

Department for Education and Department of Health (1994c) *The Education of Sick Children*, Circular No. 12/94. DH LAC (94) 10. NHSE HSG (94) 24, London: Department for Education and Department of Health.

Department for Education and Welsh Office (1992) *Drug Misuse and the Young: A Guide for the Education Services*, London: HMSO.

Department of Education and Science (1978) *Community Homes with Education*, HMI Series: Matters for Discussion 10, London: HMSO.

Department of Education and Science (1984) *The Education Welfare Service*, London: HMSO.

Department of Education and Science (1985) *Language Performance in Schools – 1982 Primary Survey Results*, London: HMSO.

Department of Education and Science (1986a) *Young People in the Eighties*, London: HMSO.

Department of Education and Science (1986b) *School Attendance and Education Welfare Services*, Circular 2/86, London: Department of Education and Science.

Department of Education and Science (1988) *Working Together for the Protection of Children from Abuse: Procedures within the Education Service*, Circular 4/88, London: Department of Education and Science.

Department of Education and Science (1989a) *Discipline in Schools: Report of the Committee of Inquiry Chaired by Lord Elton*, London, HMSO.

Department of Education and Science (1989b) *Education Observed, 13: Attendance at School*, Her Majesty's Inspectorate, London, HMSO.

Department of Education and Science (1989c) *Report by HMI Inspectors on Educating Physically Disabled Pupils*, London: Department of Education and Science.

Department of Education and Science (1989d) *A Report by HMI Inspectors: Provision for Primary Aged Pupils with Statements of Special Educational Needs in Mainstream Schools*, London: Department of Education and Science.

Department of Education and Science (1989e) *Report by HMI Inspectors on the Effectiveness of Small Special Schools*, London: Department of Education and Science.

Department of Education and Science (1990) *Educational Statistics: Schools*, London: Department of Education and Science.

Department of Education and Science (1991a) *The Parents' Charter: You and Your Children's Education*, London: Department of Education and Science.

Department of Education and Science (1991b) *The Education (Pupils' Attendance Records) Regulations, 1991*, Circular No. 11/91, London: Department of Education and Science.

Department of Education and Science (1992) *Education in Social Services Establishments: A Report by HMI*, 4/92/NS, London: Department of Education and Science.

Department of Health (1989) *The Care of Children: Principles and Practice in Regulations and Guidance*, London: HMSO.

Department of Health (1991a) *Children in the Public Care* (The Utting Report), Social Services Inspectorate, London: HMSO.

Department of Health (1991b) *The Children Act 1989: Guidance and Regulations*, vol. 7, London: HMSO.

Department of Health (1995a) *Carers (Recognition and Services) Act 1995: Policy Guidance*, London: Department of Health.

Department of Health (1995b) *Carers (Recognition and Services) Act 1995: Practice Guide*, London: Department of Health.

Department of Health (1995c) *Employment of Children: A Consultation Document*, London: Department of Health.

Department of Health (1995d) *Child Protection: Messages from the Research*, London: Department of Health.

Department of Health and Social Security (1968) *Report of the Committee on Local Authority and Allied Personal Social Services* (The Seebohm Report), Cmnd 3703, London: HMSO.

Department of Health and Social Security (1981) *Observation and Assessment: Report of a Working Party*, London: HMSO.

Digby, A. and Searby, P. (1981) *Children, School and Society in Nineteenth-Century England*, London: Macmillan.

Re DJMS – a minor – 1977 3 All ER, 582.

Doyle, C. (1995) *Helping Strategies for Child Sexual Abuse*, London: Whiting & Birch.

Driver, G. (1980) 'How West Indians do better at school (especially the girls)', *New Society*, 17 January.

Dunn, E. J. (1987) *Dealing with Non-Attendance at School – A Consideration of the Methods and Skills of Intervention Employed by the Education Welfare/Education Social Work Service: Report to the Association of Chief Education Social Workers and National Association of Social Workers in Education*, Lancaster: Department of Social Administration, University of Lancaster.

Dunn, J. and Maguire, S. (1992) 'Sibling and peer relationships in childhood', *Journal of Child Psychology and Psychiatry*, 33, 1, pp. 67–105.

Dusek, J. and Joseph, G. (1983) 'The Bases of Teacher Expectancies: A Meta-analysis', *Journal of Educational Psychology*, 75, 3, pp. 327–46.

Education (1946) *Hints for School Attendance Officers: By a Superintendent*, 12 April.

Elliott, A. (1992) *Hidden Children: A Study of Ex-Young Carers of Parents with Mental Health Problems in Leeds*, Leeds: Leeds City Council, Department of Social Services.

Elliott, M. (1985) *Preventing Child Sexual Assault*, London: Bedford Square Press.

Elliott, M. (1987) *Keeping Safe: A Practical Guide to Talking with Children*, London: Bedford Square Press.

Esposito, A. (1979) 'Sex differences in children's conversations', *Language and Speech*, 22 March, p. 213.

Essen, J., Lambert, L. and Head, J. (1976) 'School attainment of children who have been in care', *Child Care, Health and Development*, 2, pp. 339–51.

Essex CC v B (1993) 1 FLR pp. 866–82.

Evetts, J. (1996) 'The new headteacher: budgetary devolution and the work culture of secondary headship', in Pole, C. and Chawla-Duggan, R. (eds) *Reshaping Education in the 1990s: Perspectives on Secondary Schooling*, London: Falmer Press.

Fallon, M. (1992) 'Why the NCC failed to deliver', *The Times*, 23 February, p. 33.

Family Policy Studies Centre (1994) *Families in the European Union* (Special Edition), London: Family Policy Studies Centre.

Farrington of Ribbleton, Baroness (1995) 'Young carers in the education system', in *Young Carers: Back Them Up*. Report of a conference organised jointly by Community Care and Carers National Association at BMA House, London, 17 November, London: Community Care and Carers National Association.

Farrington, D. (1996) 'Later life outcomes of truants in the Cambridge study', in Berg, I. and Nursten, J. (eds) *Unwillingly to School* (4th edn), London: Gaskell.

Farrington, D. and West, D. J. (1990) 'The Cambridge study in delinquent development: a long-term follow up of 411 London males', in Kerner, H. J. and Kaiser, G. (eds) *Criminality: Personality, Behaviour and Life History*, Berlin: Springer Verlag.

Fergusson, D. and Lynskey, M. (1996) 'Adolescent Resilience to Family Adversity', *Journal of Child Psychology and Psychiatry*, 37, 3, pp. 281–292.

Fine, G. A. (1980) 'The natural history of preadolescent friendship groups', in Foot, A., Chapman, A. J. and Smith, J. R. (eds) *Friendship and Social Relations in Children*, New York: Wiley.

Finkelstein, V. (1980) *Attitudes and Disabled People: Issues for Discussion*, New York: World Rehabilitation Fund.

Finkelstein, V. (1981) 'To deny or not to deny disability', in Brechin, A., Liddiard, P. and Swain, J. (eds) *Handicap in a Social World*, London: Hodder & Stoughton in Association with the Open University.

Firth, H. (1992) 'Has recent education/social services legislation enhanced the educational opportunities of a child in "care"?' Unpublished M.Sc. dissertation, Reading: University of Reading.

Firth, H. (1995) *Children First: A Framework for Action*, Winchester: Hampshire County Council.

Fisher, D. (1996) *Pupil Referral Units*, Slough: National Foundation for Educational Research.

Fletcher, B. (1993) *Not Just a Name: The Views of Young People in Foster and Residential Care*, London: National Consumer Council and Who Cares? Trust.

Fletcher-Campbell, F. and Hall, C. (1990) *Changing Schools? Changing People? The Education of Children in Care*, Slough: National Foundation for Educational Research.

Flett, M. (1993) 'Early education in the community: a neighbourhood approach', in Ferguson, H., Gilligan, R. and Torode, R. (eds) *Surviving Childhood Adversity: Issues for Policy and Practice*, Dublin: Social Studies Press, Trinity College Dublin.

Foot, A., Chapman, A. J. and Smith, J. R. (eds) (1980) *Friendship and Social Relations in Children*, New York: Wiley.

Foster, E. (1988) 'Black girls and pastoral care', in Duncan, C. (ed.) *Pastoral Care: An Anti-Racist/Multicultural Perspective*, Oxford: Blackwell.

Fraiberg, S. (1988) *Putting the Pieces Together*, London: British Agencies for Adoption and Fostering.

Frones, I. (1995) *Among Peers. On the Meaning of Peers in the Process of Socialisation*, Oslo: Scandinavian University Press.

Furlong, V. J. (1991) 'Disaffected pupils: reconstructing the sociological perspective', *British Journal of Sociology of Education*, 12, 3, pp. 293–307.

Galton, M., Simon, B. and Coll, P. (1980) *Inside the Primary School*, London: Routledge & Kegan Paul.

Gardiner, J. (1996) 'Exclusions rise relentlessly', *Times Educational Supplement*, 8 November, p. 1.

Garner, P. (1996) *A la Récherche du Temps 'PRU': Case-Study Evidence from Off-Site and Pupil Referral Units*, paper presented at 'The Prevention and Management of Exclusion from School: An Interagency Conference', University of York, 10 July, Huddersfield:

Centre for Education Welfare Studies, University of Huddersfield and Society of Education Officers.

Gibson, A. and Barrow, J. (1986) *The Unequal Struggle*, London: CSS Publications.

Gill, D. and Monsen, J. (1996) 'The staff sharing scheme: a school-based management system for working with challenging child behaviour', in Blyth, E. and Milner, J. (eds) *Exclusion from School: Inter-professional Issues for Policy and Practice*, London: Routledge.

Gillborn, D. (1990) *'Race', Ethnicity and Education: Teaching and Learning in Multi-Ethnic Schools*, London: Unwin Hyman.

Gillborn, D. and Gipps, C. (1996) *Recent Research on the Achievements of Ethnic Minority Pupils*, London: HMSO.

Gilligan, C. (1982) *In a Different Voice*, Cambridge, MA: Harvard University Press.

Gleeson, D. (1992) 'School attendance and truancy: a socio-historical account', *Sociological Review*, 40, pp. 437–90.

Goffman, E. (1968) *Stigma: Notes on the Management of a Spoiled Identity*, New Jersey: Prentice Hall.

Goldstein, H. and Sammons, P. (1995) *The Influence of Secondary and Junior Schools on Sixteen Year Examination Performance: A Cross-Classified Multilevel Analysis*, London: Institute of Education.

Graham, H. (1993) 'Caring for children in poverty', in Ferguson, H., Gilligan, R. and Torode, R. (eds) *Surviving Childhood Adversity: Issues for Policy and Practice*, Dublin: Social Studies Press, Trinity College Dublin.

Graham, J. (1992) *Family, School and Community: Towards a Social Crime Prevention Agenda*, Swindon: Crime Concern.

Graham, J. and Bowling, B. (1995) *Young People and Crime: Home Office Research Study 145*, London: Home Office.

Gray, J. (1994) 'The quality of schooling: frameworks for judgement', in Moon, B. and Shelton Mayes, A. (eds) *Teaching and Learning in the Secondary School*, London: Routledge (in association with the Open University).

Gray, J. and Jesson, D. (1990) *Truancy in Secondary Schools amongst Fifth Year Pupils*, Sheffield: University of Sheffield.

Gray, G., Smith, A. and Rutter, M. (1980) 'School attendance and the first year of employment', in Hersov, L. and Berg, I. (eds) *Out of School: Modern Perspectives in Truancy and School Refusal*, Chichester: John Wiley.

Green, D. (1993) *Reinventing Civil Society: The Rediscovery of Welfare Without Politics*, Choice in Welfare Series No 17, London: Institute for Economic Affairs.

Green, F. (1980) 'On becoming a truant – the social administrative process in non-attendance'. Unpublished MA thesis, Cranfield: Cranfield Institute of Technology.

Greenberger, E. and Steinberg, L. (1986) *When Teenagers Work: The Psychological and Social Costs of Adolescent Employment*, New York: Basic Books Inc.

Grenville, M. (1988) 'Compulsory school attendance and the child's wishes', *Journal of Social Welfare Law*, 1, pp. 4–20.

Grimshaw, R. and Berridge, D. (1994) *Educating Disruptive Children: Placement and Progress in Residential Special Schools for Emotional and Behavioural Difficulties*, London: National Children's Bureau.

Hackett, G. (1992) 'Brent seeks ruling on exclusions', *Times Educational Supplement*, 17 July, p. 2.

Hagedorn, J. (1992) *Observer Schools Report*, 18 October, p. 4.

Hainsworth, G. (1996) 'Working with boys', in Cavanagh, K. and Cree, V. E. (eds) *Working with Men: Feminism and Social Work*, London and New York: Routledge.

Halford, P. (1994) 'The Education Welfare/Education Social Work Service in England and Wales: A Critique of its Organisation and Role'. Unpublished M.Phil. thesis, Southampton: University of Southampton.

Hallett, C. and Birchall, E. (1992) *Co-ordination and Child Protection: A Review of the Literature*, Edinburgh: HMSO.

Hamilton, S. and O'Reilly, J. (1997) 'Tory school opt-out drive hits buffers', *Sunday Times*, 16 March, p. 12.

Hart, S. (1977) *Violence, Disruption and Vandalism in Schools – A Summary of the Research*, London: National Children's Bureau.

Hawkins, J., Catalano, R. and Miller, J. (1992) 'Risk and protective factors for alcohol and other drug problems in adolescence and early adulthood: implications of substance abuse prevention', *Psychological Bulletin*, 112, pp. 64–105.

Haywood, C. and Mac an Ghaill, M. (1996) 'Schooling masculinities', in Mac an Ghaill, M. (ed.) *Understanding Masculinities*, Buckingham: Open University Press.

Hearn, J. (1996) 'Men's known violence to women: historical, everyday and theoretical constructions by men', in Fawcett, B., Featherstone, B. Hearn, J. and Toft, C. (eds) *Violence and Gender Relations: Theories and Interventions*, London: Sage.

Heath, A., Colton, M. and Aldgate, J. (1989) 'The educational progress of children in and out of care', *British Journal of Social Work*, 19, 6, pp. 447–60.

Heath, A., Colton, M. and Aldgate, J. (1994) 'Failure to escape: a longitudinal study of foster-children's educational attainment', *British Journal of Social Work*, 24, 3, pp. 241–59.

Heward, C. and Lloyd-Smith, M. (1990) 'Assessing the impact of legislation on special education policy – an historical analysis', *Journal of Education Policy*, 5, pp. 21–36.

Hibbett, A. and Fogelman, K. (1990) 'Future lives of truants in family formation and health-related benefits', *British Journal of Educational Psychology*, 60, pp. 171–9.

Hibbett, A., Fogelman, K. and Manor, O. (1990) 'Occupation and outcomes of truancy', *British Journal of Educational Psychology*, 60, pp. 23–36.

Higgins, G. (1994) 'Hammersmith Women's Aid Childwork Development Project', in Mullender, A. and Morley, R. (eds) *Children Living with Domestic Violence: Putting Men's Abuse of Women on the Child Care Agenda*, London: Whiting & Birch.

Hinchliffe, D. (1995) Parliamentary Debates, 258, 463, 21 April.

HMI (1978a) *Truancy and Behaviour Problems in Some Urban Schools*, London: Department of Education and Science.

HMI (1978b) *Behavioural Units. A Survey of Special Units for Pupils with Behavioural Problems*, London: Department of Education and Science.

HMI (1979) *Aspects of Secondary Education: A Survey of HM Inspectors of Schools*, London: Department of Education and Science.

HMSO (1978) *Special Educational Needs. Report of the Committee of Enquiry Into the Education of Handicapped Children and Young People* (The Warnock Report), Cmnd 7212, London: HMSO.

HMSO (1993) *Children Act 1989: A Report by the Secretaries of State for Health and for Wales on the Children Act 1989 in pursuance of their duties under Section 83(6) of the Act,* Cm 2144, London: HMSO.

HMSO (1994) *The UK's First Report to the UN Committee on the Rights of the Child*, London: HMSO.

Hofkins D. (1990) 'Pressed to alter rights on special needs', *Times Educational Supplement,* 26 October.

Holmes, G. (1989) *Truancy and Social Welfare*, Manchester: Boys and Girls Welfare Society/Manchester Free Press.

Home Office, Department of Health, Department of Education and Science and Welsh Office (1991) *Working Together Under the Children Act: A Guide for Arrangements for Inter-agency Co-operation for the Protection of Children from Abuse*, London: HMSO.

House of Commons (1984) *Second Report from the Social Services Select Committee: Children in Care*, London: HMSO.

House of Commons (1993) *Third Report from the Education Committee: Meeting Special Educational Needs: Statements of Needs and Provision*, London: HMSO.

House of Commons (1995) *Performance in City Schools: Minutes of Evidence*, Education Committee, 1 March, London: HMSO.

Hughes, J. M. (1984) *The Best Years?* Aberdeen: Aberdeen University Press.

Hughes, M. and Lloyd, E. (1996) 'Young people: stakeholders in the educational system', in Roberts, H. and Sachdev, D. (eds) *Young People's Social Attitudes: Having Their Say – The Views of 12–19 Year Olds*, Barkingside: Barnardos.

Hullin, R. (1985) 'The Leeds truancy project', *Justice of the Peace*, 149, pp. 488–90.

Hullin, R. (1988) 'The juvenile court and non-attendance at school: a reply to Messrs Blyth and Milner', *Justice of the Peace*, 152, pp. 247–50.

Imich, A. (1994) 'Exclusions from school: current trends and issues', *Educational Research*, 36, 1, Spring, pp. 3–11.

Ingleby, D. (1984) 'Professionals as socialisers: the "psy complex"', in Aplин, N. and Oull, M. T. (eds) *Research in Law, Deviance and Social Control*, London: JAI Press.

Inner London Education Authority (1990) *Differences in Examination Performance* (RS1277/990), London: ILEA Research and Statistics Branch.

Jackson, S. (1987) *The Education of Children in Care*: Bristol Papers in Applied Social Studies, Bristol: University of Bristol.

Jackson, S. (1988–9) 'Residential care and education', *Children and Society*, 4, pp. 335–50.

Jackson, S. (1989) 'Education of children in care', in Kahan, B. (ed.) *Child Care Research, Policy and Practice*, London: Hodder & Stoughton in association with the Open University.

Jackson, S. (1994) 'Educating children in residential and foster care', *Oxford Review of Education*, 20, 3, pp. 267–79.

Jackson, S. (1995) 'Education in care: not somebody else's problem', *Professional Social Work*, November, pp. 12–13.

Jackson, S. and Cairns, B. (1986) 'The educational experiences of children in care', unpublished report to the Department of Health and Social Security, Bristol: University of Bristol.

Jaffe, P., Wolfe, D. and Wilson, S. K. (1990) *Children of Battered Women*, Newbury Park, CA: Sage.

Johnston, P. (1994) 'Tory taxes "cost poor £3 a week"', *Daily Telegraph*, 9 February, p. 9.

Jones, C. (1992) 'Fertility of the over thirties', *Population Trends*, 67, pp. 10–16.

Kadushin, A. and Martin, J. A. (1981) *Child Abuse: An Interactional Event*, New York: Columbia University Press.

Kahan, B. (1985) 'Learning to lose', *Social Work Today*, 29 April, p. 21.

Kahn, T. J. and Chambers, H. (1991) 'Assessing reoffence risk with juvenile sex offenders', *Child Welfare*, LXX, 3.

Kavanagh, S. (1989) 'Split decisions', *Times Educational Supplement*, 6 October, p. 26.

Kazi, M. and Wilson, J. (1996) 'Applying single-case evaluation in social work', *British Journal of Social Work*, 26, 2, pp. 699–717.

Keith, L. and Morris, J. (1995) 'Easy targets: a disability rights perspective on the "children as carers" debate', *Critical Social Policy*, 44/45, pp. 36–7.

Kelly, A. (1981) *The Missing Half: Girls and Science Education*, Manchester: Manchester University Press.

Kelly, A. (1988) 'Ethnic differences: science choice, attitudes and achievement in Britain', *British Educational Research Journal*, 14, 2, pp. 113–26.

Kelly, L. (1992) 'The connections between disability and child abuse: a review of the research evidence', *Child Abuse Review*, 1, pp. 157–67.

Kelly, L. (1994) 'The interconnectedness of domestic violence and child abuse: challenges for research and practice', in Mullender, A. and Morley, R. (eds) *Children Living with Domestic Violence: Putting Men's Abuse of Women on the Child Care Agenda*, London: Whiting & Birch.

Kelly, L., Regan, L. and Burton, S. (1991) *An Exploratory Study of the Prevalence of Sexual Abuse in a Sample of 16–21 Year Olds*, London: CSAU, North London Polytechnic.

Kelly, L., Regan, I. and Burton, S. (1993) 'Beyond victim to survivor: the implications of knowledge about children's resistance and avoidance strategies', in Ferguson, H., Gilligan, R. and Torode, R. (eds) *Surviving Childhood Adversity: Issues for Policy and Practice*, Dublin: Social Studies Press, Trinity College Dublin.

Kelly, N. and Milner, J. (1996) 'Decision making in child protection', *Child Abuse Review*, pp. 91–102.

Kennedy, D. (1996) 'Mental illness will "strike 40% of children"', *The Times*, 2 December, p. 6.

Kennedy, M. (1995) 'Rights for children who are disabled', in Franklin, B. (ed.) *The Handbook of Children's Rights*, London: Routledge.

Kennedy, M. and Gordon, R. (eds) (1993) *Abuse and Children who are Disabled*, London: Department of Health.

Keys, W. and Fernandes, C. (1990) *A Survey of School Governing Bodies*, Slough: National Foundation for Educational Research.

King's Fund Centre (undated) *Young Carers in Black and Minority Ethnic Communities: Workshop Day Report*, London: King's Fund Centre.

Knapp, M., Bryson, D. and Lewis, J. (1985) *The Objectives of Child Care and their Attainment over a Twelve Month Period for a Cohort of New Admissions, The Suffolk Cohort Study, Discussion Paper 373*, Canterbury: PSSRU, University of Kent at Canterbury.

Knight, K. (1996) 'Girls are sent home for wearing wrong trousers', *The Times*, 30 November, p. 11.

Lavalette, M., Hobbs, S., Lindsay, S. and McKechnie, J. (1995) 'Child employment in Britain: policy, myth and reality', *Youth & Policy*, 47, pp. 1–15.

Leach, P. (1994) *Children First*, London: Michael Joseph.

Learmonth, J. (1995) *More Willingly to School? An Independent Evaluation of the Truancy and Disaffected Pupils GEST Programme*, London: Department for Education and Employment.

Lee, T. (1990) *Carving out the Cash for Schools: LMS and the New ERA of Education*, Bath Social Policy Paper no. 17, Bath: University of Bath.

Lees, S. (1986) *Losing Out: Sexuality and Adolescent Girls*, Hutchinson, London.

Levy, A. and Kahan, B. (1991) *The Pindown Experience and the Protection of Children. The Report on the Staffordshire Child Care Enquiry*, Stafford: Staffordshire County Council.

Lewis, E. (1995) *Truancy: The Partnership Approach*, Stoke on Trent: Smith Davis Press.

Licht, B. G. and Dweck, C. S. (1983) 'Sex differences in science achievement orientations: consequences for academic choices and attainments', in Marland, M. (ed.) *Sex Differentiation and Schooling*, London: Heinemann.

London Borough of Brent (1985) *A Child in Trust: Report of the Panel of Inquiry into the Circumstances surrounding the Death of Jasmine Beckford*, London: London Borough of Brent.

London Borough of Enfield (1995) *Young Carers and Education: Research and Development Project 1994/5*, Enfield: London Borough of Enfield.

London Borough of Greenwich (1987) *A Child in Mind: Protection of Children in a Responsible Society: The Report of the Commission of Inquiry into the Circumstances surrounding the Death of Kimberley Carlile*, London: HMSO.

London Borough of Lambeth (1985) *Whose Child? The Report of the Panel Appointed to Inquire into the Death of Tyra Henry*, London: London Borough of Lambeth.

Lonsdale, S. (1990) *Women and Disability*, London: Macmillan.

McAdoo, H. P. and McAdoo, J. L. (1985) *Black Children: Social, Educational and Parental Environments*, London: Sage.

Mac an Ghaill, M. (1988) *Young, Gifted and Black*, Milton Keynes: Open University Press.

Mac an Ghaill, M. (1994) *The Making of Men*, Milton Keynes: Open University Press.

McCalman, J. (1990) *The Forgotten People: A Study of Carers in Three Minority Ethnic Communities*, London: King's Fund Centre.

Macdonald, I., Bhavnani, R., Khan, L. and John, G. (1989) *Murder in the Playground: The Burnage Report*, London: Longsight Press.

McKeown, P., Donnelly, C. and Osborne, B. (1996) 'School governing bodies in Northern Ireland: responses to local management of schools', in Pole, C. and Chawla-Duggan, R. (eds) *Reshaping Education in the 1990s: Perspectives on Secondary Schooling*, London: Falmer Press.

Maclure, J. S. (ed.) (1965) *Educational Documents, England and Wales 1816–1963*, London: Chapman & Hall.

McManus, M. (1995) *Troublesome Behaviour in the Classroom: Meeting Individual Needs*, London: Routledge.

MacMillan, K. (1977) *Education Welfare: Strategy and Structure*, London: Longman.

McParlin, P. (1996) 'Children "looked after" (in care) – implications for educational psychologists', *Educational Psychology in Practice*, 12, 2, pp. 112–17.

McPherson, A. (1992) *Measuring Added Value in Schools. National Commission on Education Briefing Paper*, London: National Commission on Education.

Magistrates' Association (1994) *Notes of a meeting held on 28 October 1994 between the Magistrates' Association and representatives of agencies involved with prosecution of parents under the Education Acts*, London: Magistrates' Association.

Maher, P. (1987) *Child Abuse: The Educational Perspective*, Oxford: Basil Blackwell.

Mahon, A. and Higgins, J. (1995) '. . . *A life of our own'. Young Carers: An Evaluation of Three RHA Funded Projects on Merseyside*, Manchester: Health Services Management Unit, Manchester University.

Mahoney, P. (1985) *School for the Boys*, London: Hutchinson.

Manning, M., Heron, J. and Marshall, T. (1978) 'Styles of hostility and social interactions at nursery school and at home', in Hersov, L. (ed.) *Aggression and Antisocial Behaviour in Childhood and Adolescence*, Oxford, Pergamon.

Marchant, R. and Page, M. (1993) *Bridging the Gap: Child Protection with Children with Multiple Disabilities*, London: NSPCC.

Mardon, J. (1996) 'A parenting course for young men', in Newburn, T. and Mair, G. (eds) *Working with Men*, Lyme Regis: Russell House Publishing.

Margolin, L. (1993) 'In their parents' absence: sexual abuse in child care', *Violence Update*, 3, 9, pp. 1, 2, 4, 8.

Marshall, W. (1996) 'Professionals, children and power', in Blyth, E. and Milner, J. (eds) *Exclusion from School: Inter-professional Issues for Policy and Practice*, London: Routledge.

Martin, J. and White, A. (1988) *The Financial Circumstances of Disabled Adults Living in Private Households*, London: HMSO.

Mayes, G. M., Currie, E. F., Macleod, L., Gillies, J. B. and Warden, D. A. (1992) *Child Sexual Abuse: A Review of the Literature and Educational Material*, Edinburgh: Scottish Academic Press.

Measor, L. and Woods, P. (1984) *Changing Schools: Pupils' Perspectives on Transfer to a Comprehensive*, Milton Keynes: Open University Press.

Melotte, C. J. (1979) 'The placement decision', *Adoption and Fostering*, 95, 1, pp. 55–62.

Meltzer, H., Smyth, M. and Robus, N. (1989) *Disabled Children: Services, Transport and Education*, London: OPCS.

Middleton, L. (1996) *Making a Difference: Social Work with Disabled Children*, Birmingham: Venture Press.

Millham, S., Bullock, R. and Hosie, K. (1980) *Learning to Care: The Training of Staff for Residential Social Work with Young People*, Aldershot: Gower.

Millham, S. Bullock, R., Hosie, K. and Haak, M. (1986) *Lost in Care*, Aldershot: Gower.

Milner, J. (1993) 'Avoiding violent men: the gendered nature of child protection policy and practice', in Ferguson, H., Gilligan, R. and Torode, R. (eds) *Surviving Childhood Adversity: Issues for Policy and Practice*, Dublin: Social Studies Press, Trinity College Dublin.

Milner, J. (1996) 'Men's resistance to social workers', in Fawcett, B., Featherstone, B., Hearn, J. and Toft, C. (eds) *Violence and Gender Relations*, London: Sage.

Milner, J. and Blyth, E. (1988) *Coping with Child Sexual Abuse. a Guide for Teachers*, York: Longman.

Mintel (1994) *British Lifestyles 1994*, London: Mintel.

Mirza, H. S. (1992) *Young, Female and Black*, London: Routledge.

Mitchell, L. (1996) 'The effects of waiting time on excluded children', in Blyth, E. and Milner, J. (eds) *School Exclusions: Interprofessional Issues for Policy and Practice*, London: Routledge.

Mongon, D. (1988) 'Behaviour units, maladjustment and student control', in Slee, R. (ed.) *Discipline and Control: A Curriculum Perspective*, Melbourne: Macmillan.

Montgomery, J. (1996) 'Truants' parents feel the force of law', *Times Educational Supplement*, 10 May, p. 5.

Moore, D. and Davenport, S. (1990) 'Choice: the new improved sorting machine', in Boyd, W. L. and Walberg, H. J. (eds) *Choice in Education: Potential and Problems*, Berkeley, CA: McCutchan.

Morley, R. and Mullender, A. (1994) 'Domestic violence and children: what do we know from research?' in Mullender, A. and Morley, R. (eds) *Children Living with Domestic Violence: Putting Men's Abuse of Women on the Child Care Agenda*, London: Whiting & Birch.

Morris, J. (ed.) (1989) *Able Lives: Women's Experience of Paralysis*, London: The Women's Press.

Morris, J. (1991) *Pride Against Prejudice: Transforming Attitudes to Disability*, London: The Women's Press.

Morris, J. (1995) *Gone Missing: Research and Policy Review of Disabled Children Living Away from the Families*, London: The Who Cares? Trust.

Mortimore, P., Sammons, P., Stoll, L., Lewis, D. and Ecob, R. (1988a) *School Matters? The Junior Years*, London: Open Books.

Mortimore, P., Sammons, P., Stoll, L., Lewis, D. and Ecob, R. (1988b) 'The effects of school membership on pupils' educational outcomes', *Research Papers in Education*, 3, 1, pp. 3–26.

Mortimore, P., Sammons, P., Stoll, L., Lewis, D. and Ecob, R. (1994) 'Teacher expectations', in Moon, B. and Shelton Mayes, A. (eds) *Teaching and Learning in the Secondary School*, London: Routledge (in association with the Open University).

Mullender, A. (1994) 'School-based work: education for prevention', in Mullender, A. and Morley, R. (eds) *Children Living with Domestic Violence: Putting Men's Abuse of Women on the Child Care Agenda*, London: Whiting & Birch.

Murphy, P. (1994) 'Assessment and gender', in Moon, B. and Shelton Mayes, A. (eds) *Teaching and Learning in the Secondary School*, London: Routledge (in association with the Open University).

National Association for the Care and Resettlement of Offenders (1997) *A New Three Rs for Young Offenders: Responsibility, Restoration and Reintegration. Towards a New Strategy for Children Who Offend.* London: NACRO.

National Association of Social Workers in Education (1994) *Young Carers.* Policy Document No 15.

National Association of Social Workers in Education (1996) *NASWE Data Book*, NASWE.

National Commission of Inquiry into the Prevention of Child Abuse (1996) *Childhood Matters*, London: The Stationery Office.

National Union of Teachers (1992) *Survey on Pupils' Exclusions: Information from LEAs*, May, London: NUT.

NCH: Action for Children (1994) Press release: *The Workhouse Diet and the Cost of Feeding a Child Today*, 1 February.

Normington, J. (1996) 'Exclusion from school: the role of outside agencies', in Blyth, E. and Milner, J. (eds) *School Exclusions: Interprofessional Issues for Policy and Practice*, London: Routledge.

Northern Ireland Research Team (1991) *Child Sexual Abuse in Northern Ireland*, Belfast: Greystone.

Nowicka, H. (1993) 'Fears over "Truant Watch"', *Independent on Sunday*, 28 November, p. 2.

Re O (A Minor) (Care Order: Education Procedure) (1992) 2 FLR FD pp. 8–13.

O'Callaghan, D. and Print, B. (1994) 'Adolescent sexual abusers: research, assessment and treatment', in Morrison, T., Erooga, M. and Becket, R. C. (eds) *Sexual Offending Against Children*, London: Routledge.

O'Connor, M., Hales, E., Davies, J. and Tomlinson, S. (1997) *Hackney Downs: The School that Dared to Fight*, Basingstoke: Falmer Press.

OECD (1995) *Income Distribution in OECD Countries*, OECD: Paris.

OFSTED (1993a) *Education for Disaffected Pupils: 1990–1992.* A report from the Office of Her Majesty's Chief Inspector of Schools (Ref: 1/93/NS). London: HMSO.

OFSTED (1993b) *Achieving Good Behaviour in Schools.* A report from the Office of Her Majesty's Chief Inspector of Schools. London: HMSO.

OFSTED (1995a) *Access, Achievement and Attendance in Secondary Schools*, London: OFSTED.

OFSTED (1995b) *The Challenge for Education Welfare*: A report from the Office of Her Majesty's Chief Inspector of Schools (Ref 17/95/NS), London: OFSTED.

OFSTED (1995c) *Pupil Referral Units: The First Twelve Inspections.* A report from the Office of Her Majesty's Chief Inspector of Schools, London: OFSTED.

OFSTED (1996a) *The Ridings School.* A report from the Office of Her Majesty's Chief Inspector of Schools (Ref: 82/96/SZ), London: OFSTED.

OFSTED (1996b) *Exclusions from Secondary Schools 1995/6.* A report from the Office of Her Majesty's Chief Inspector of Schools, London: The Stationery Office.

O'Keeffe, D. (1994) *Truancy in English Secondary Schools*, London: HMSO.

Oliver, M. (1983) *Social Work with Disabled People*, Basingstoke: Macmillan.

Oliver, M. (1990) *The Politics of Disablement*, Basingstoke: Macmillan.

Olsen, R. (1996) 'Young carers: challenging the facts and politics of research into children and caring', *Disability and Society*, 11, 1, pp. 41–54.

Olweus, D. (1979) *Aggression in Schools*, New York: Wiley.

Olweus, D. (1993) *Bullying at School: What We Know and What We Can Do*, Oxford: Basil Blackwell.

O'Neill, A. (1988) *Young Carers: The Tameside Research*, Ashton-under-Lyne: Tameside Metropolitan Borough Council.

O'Neill, A. and Platt, C. (1992) *Towards a Strategy for Carers*, Tameside: Young Carers Policy Research Unit, Ashton-under-Lyne: Tameside Metropolitan Borough Council.

OPCS (1992) *General Household Survey: Carers in 1990*, OPCS Monitor SS 92/2, London: HMSO.

O'Reilly, J. (1996a) 'Teenagers sue schools for bad exam results', *Sunday Times*, 1 December, p. 1.

O'Reilly, J. (1996b) 'Special schools fail to help needy pupils', *Sunday Times*, 24 November, p. 9.

Page, R. (1988) *Report on the Initial Survey Investigating the Number of Young Carers in Sandwell Secondary Schools*, West Bromwich: Sandwell Metropolitan Borough Council.

Parker, G. (1993) *With this Body: Caring and Disability in Marriage*, Buckingham: Open University Press.

Parker, G. (1994) *Where Next for Research on Carers?* Leicester: Nuffield Community Care Studies Unit, Leicester University.

Parker, R. A. (1988) 'Residential care for children', in Sinclair, I. (ed.) *Residential Care: The Research Reviewed. Literature Surveys Commissioned by the Independent Review of Residential Care* (The Wagner Report), London: NISW/HMSO.

Parker, R. A., Ward, H., Jackson, S., Aldgate, J. and Wedge, P. (1991) *Looking after Children: Assessing Outcomes in Child Care*, London: HMSO.

Parsons, C., Benns, L., Hailes, J. and Howlett, K. (1994) *Excluding Primary School Children*, London: Family Policy Studies Centre.

Parsons, C., Hailes, J., Howlett, K., Davies, A. and Driscoll, P. (1995) *National Survey of Local Education Authorities' Policies and Procedures for the Identification of, and Provision for, Children who are Out of School by Reason of Exclusion or Otherwise: Final Report to the Department for Education*, Canterbury: Christ Church College.

Patten, J. (1992) reported in *Education*, 179, 19, 8 May, p. 370.

Patten, J. (1993) BBC Radio 4 News, 17 November.

Pearson, G. (1983) *Hooligans: A History of Respectable Fears*, London: Macmillan.

Peters, R. D., McMahon, R. J. and Quinsey, V. L. (eds) (1992) *Aggression and Violence through the Life Span*, London: Sage.

Petre, J. (1994) 'Tougher fines for parents of truants urged', *Sunday Telegraph*, 3 July, p. 8.

Phoenix, A. (1991) *Young Mothers*, London: Polity Press.

Pilling, D. and Kelmer Pringle, M. (1978) *Controversial Issues in Child Development*, London: Paul Elek.

Platt, A. (1969) 'The rise of the child saving movement', *Annals of the American Academy*, January, p. 381.

Pond, C. and Searle, A. (1991) *The Hidden Army: Children at Work in the 1990s*. Low Pay Unit Pamphlet 55, London: Low Pay Unit.

Power, S., Fitz, J. and Halpin, D. (1994) 'Parents, pupils and grant-maintained schools', *British Educational Research Journal*, 20, 2, pp. 209–26.

Power, S., Halpin, D. and Fitz, J. (1996) 'The grant-maintained schools policy: the English experience of educational self-governance', in Pole, C. and Chawla-Duggan, R. (eds) *Reshaping Education in the 1990s: Perspectives on Secondary Schooling*, London: Falmer Press.

Pyke, N. (1990) 'Cuts blamed for rise in special needs referrals', *Times Educational Supplement*, 21 September, p. 19.

Pyke, N. (1996) 'Expenditure time bomb fears over special help', *Times Educational Supplement*, 29 November, p. 3.

Quality in Education Centre for Research and Consultancy (1995) *The Truancy File*, Glasgow: University of Strathclyde.

Rampton, A. (1981) *West Indian Children in Our Schools* (The Rampton Report), Cmnd 8273, London: HMSO.

Ranson, S. (1984) 'Towards a tertiary tripartism: new codes of social control and the 17+', in Broadfoot, P. (ed.) *Selection, Certification and Control*, Lewes: Falmer Press.

Ranson, S. (1990) 'From 1944 to 1988: education, citizenship and democracy', in Flude, M. and Hammer, M. (eds) *The Education Reform Act 1988: Its Origins and Implications*, Falmer Press, Lewes.

Reder, P., Duncan, S. and Gary, M. (1993) *Beyond Blame: Child Abuse Tragedies Revisited*, London: Routledge.

Reid, K. (1985) *Truancy and School Absenteeism*, London: Hodder & Stoughton.

Reynolds, D. (1996) 'School factors', in Berg, I. and Nursten, J. (eds) *Unwillingly to School* (4th edn), London: Gaskell.

Reynolds, D. and Cuttance, P. (eds) (1992) *School Effectiveness: Research, Policy and Practice*, London: Cassell.

Rieser, R. (1995) 'Developing a whole-school approach to inclusion: making the most of the Code and the 1993 Act: a personal view', in National Children's Bureau *Schools Special Educational Needs Policies Pack: Discussion Papers III*, London: National Children's Bureau.

Robertson, I. (1996) 'Legal Problems', in Berg, I. and Nursten, J. (eds) *Unwillingly to School* (4th edn), London: Gaskell.

Robinson, M. (1978) *Schools and Social Work*, London: Routledge & Kegan Paul.

Rodgers, M. (forthcoming) *School Attendance – The Legislative Powers to Enforce and the Effectiveness of the Remedies*.

Rogers, R. (1986) *Caught in the Act*, London: Centre for Studies on Integration in Education.

Romans, S., Martin, J., Anderson, J., O'Shea, M. and Mullen, P. (1995) 'Factors that mediate between child sexual abuse and adult psychological outcome', *Psychological Medicine*, 25, pp. 127–42.

Rose, N. (1985) *The Psychological Complex*, London: Routledge & Kegan Paul.

Rosenthal, H. (1993) 'Friendship groups: an approach to helping friendless children', *Educational Psychology in Practice*, 9, 2, pp. 112–20.

Rosenthal, R. and Jacobsen, L. (1968) *Pygmalion in the Classroom*, New York: Rinehart & Winston.

Royal Association for Disability and Rehabilitation (1992) 'Report shows education act is failing disabled children', *RADAR Bulletin*, October.

Rubenstein, D. (1969) *School Attendance in London 1870–1904*, Hull: Hull University Press.

Russell, P. (1995) 'Policy and diversity: addressing values and principles when developing a school policy for children with special educational needs', in National Children's Bureau *Schools Special Educational Needs Policies Pack: Discussion Papers I*, London: National Children's Bureau.

Rutter, M. (1991a) 'Pathways from childhood to adult life: the role of schooling', *Pastoral Care in Education*, 9, 3, pp. 3–10.

Rutter, M. (1991b) 'Services for children with emotional disorders', *Young Minds Newsletter*, 9, October, pp. 1–5.

Rutter, M. and Rutter, M. (1993) *Developing Minds: Challenge and Continuity across the Life Span*, Harmondsworth: Penguin.

Rutter, M., Maughan, B., Mortimore, P. and Ouston, J. (1979) *Fifteen Thousand Hours: Secondary Schools and their Effects on Children*, London: Open Books.

Rutter, M., Maughan, B., and Ouston, J. (1986) 'The study of school effectiveness', in van der Wolf, J. C. and Hox, J. J. (eds) *Kwaliteit van Ondertings in het Geding*, Lisse: Swets & Zeitlinger.

Ryan, G. and Lane, S. (eds) (1991) *Juvenile Sexual Offending: Its Causes, Consequences and Connections*, Lexington, MA: Lexington Books.

Sage, G. (1993) *Child Abuse and the Children Act: A Critical Analysis of the Teacher's Rôle*, London: Association of Teachers and Lecturers Publications.

Sammons, P., Hillman, J. and Mortimore, P. (1995) *Key Characteristics of Effective Schools: A Review of School Effectiveness research*, London: OFSTED.

Samson, A. and Hart, G. (1995) 'A whole school approach to the management of pupil behaviour', in Farrell, P. (ed.) *Children with Emotional and Behavioural Difficulties: Strategies for Assessment and Intervention*, London: The Falmer Press.

Sandwell Caring for Carers Project (1989) *Child Carers Report*, West Bromwich: Sandwell Metropolitan Borough Council.

Schachar, M., Rutter, M. and Smith, A. (1981) 'The characteristics of situationally and pervasively hyperactive children', *Journal of Child Psychology and Psychiatry*, 22, pp. 375–92.

Scott-Clark, C. and Burke, J. (1996) 'Who, me?' *Sunday Times*, 19 May, p. 10.

Scott-Clark, C. and Syal, R. (1996) 'Running Wild', *Sunday Times*, 28 April, p. 12.

Scottish Council for Research on Education (1992) *Truancy and Attendance in Scottish Secondary Schools,* Spotlights no. 38, Edinburgh: Scottish Council for Research on Education.

Scottish Office Education Department (1977) *Truancy and Indiscipline in Scotland* (The Pack Report), Edinburgh: HMSO.

Scottish Office Education Department (1995) *Parents' Charter: Information for Parents – Authorised and Unauthorised Absence*, Circular 1/95, Edinburgh: Scottish Office Education Department.

Secondary Heads Association (1992) *Excluded from School: A Survey of Secondary School Suspensions,* Bristol: SHA.

Secretary of State (1988) *Report of the Inquiry into Child Abuse in Cleveland*, London: HMSO.

Segal, J. and Simkins, J. (1993) *My Mum Needs Me: Helping Children with Ill or Disabled parents*, Harmondsworth: Penguin.

Segal, L. (1990) *Slow Motion: Changing Masculinities, Changing Men*, London: Virago.

Shephard, G. (1994) quoted in *The Times School Report*, 22 November, p. 1.

Sim *v* Rotherham Metropolitan BC and other actions (1986) 3 All ER, pp. 387–416.

Simpson, P. (1990) 'Education for disabled children – today and tomorrow', *Contact*, 64, Summer, pp. 9–11.

Sinclair, R. (1994) *The Education of Children in Need*, paper presented at the Third International Child Care Conference, Birmingham, 22 March.

Sinclair, R., Garnett, L., Beecham, J. and Berridge, D. (1993) *Social Work and Assessment with Adolescents*, London: National Children's Bureau.

Sinclair, R., Grimshaw, R. and Garnett, L. (1994) 'The education of children in need: the impact of the Education Reform Act 1988, the Education Act 1993 and the Children Act 1989', *Oxford Review of Education*, 20, 3, pp. 281–92.

Sletta, O., Valås, H. and Skaalvik, E. (1996) 'Peer relations, loneliness and self-perceptions in school-aged children', *British Journal of Educational Psychology*, 66, 4, pp. 431–46.

Slukin, A. (1981) *Growing up in the Playground*, London: Routledge & Kegan Paul.

Smith, D. and Tomlinson, S. (1989) *The School Effect: A Study of Multiracial Comprehensives*, London: Policy Studies Institute

Smith, P. and Sharpe, S. (1994) *School Bullying: Insights and Perspectives*, London: Routledge.

Smith, S. (1989) 'Should they be kept apart?' *Times Educational Supplement*, 18 July, p. 36.

Social Services Inspectorate (1994) *Services to Disabled Children and their Families: Report of the National Inspection of Services to Disabled Children and their Families*, London: HMSO.

Social Services Inspectorate (1995a) *Young Carers*, CI (95) 12, 28 April, London: Department of Health.

Social Services Inspectorate (1995b) *Young Carers: Something to Think About. Report of Four SSI Workshops, May–July 1995*, London: Department of Health.

Social Services Inspectorate (1996) *Young Carers: Making a Start*, London: Department of Health.

Social Services Inspectorate and OFSTED (1995) *The Education of Children who are Looked After by Local Authorities*, London: Department of Health and OFSTED.

Solihull Metropolitan Borough Council (1992) *Legal Enforcement – School Attendance*, Report by Director of Education, 8 January, Solihull: Solihull Metropolitan Borough Council.

Southgate, V. (1981) *Extended Beginning Reading*, London: Schools Council.

Spencer, D. (1982) 'Staying on helps blacks to exam success', *Times Educational Supplement*, 8 October, p. 5.

Stein, M. (1986) *Living Out of Care*, Barnardos: Ilford.

Stein, M. (1994) 'Leaving care, education and career trajectories', *Oxford Review of Education*, 20, 3, pp. 349–60.

Stein, M. and Carey, K. (1983) *Leaving Care*, Blackwell: Oxford.

Stephenson, M. (1996) 'Cities in schools: a new approach for excluded children and young people', in Blyth, E. and Milner, J. (eds) *Exclusion from School: Inter-professional Issues for Policy and Practice*, London: Routledge.

Stephenson, P. and Smith, D. (1987) 'Anatomy of a playground bully', *Education*, Sept., pp. 236–7.

Stevenson, J. and Hague, L. (1954) *Handbook of Child Care Law*, London: Pitman.

Stirling, M. (1996) 'Government policy and disadvantaged children', in Blyth, E. and Milner, J. (eds) *Exclusion from School: Inter-professional Issues for Policy and Practice*, London: Routledge.

Stoll, P. A. and O'Keeffe, D. J. (1989) *Officially Present: An Investigation into Post-Registration Truancy in Nine Maintained Secondary Schools*, London: Institute of Economic Affairs.

Sudermann, M., Jaffe, P. G., Hastings, E. with Watson, L., Greer, G. and Lehmann, P. (1994) *ASAP: A School Based Anti-violence Programme*, London, Ontario: London Family Court Clinic.

Swann, Lord (1985) *Education for All: Final Report of the Committee of*

Inquiry into the Education of Children from Ethnic Minority Groups (The Swann Report) Cmnd 9453, London: HMSO.

Tattum, D. (1993) *Understanding and Managing Bullying*, London, Heinemann.

Taylor, C., Roberts, J. and Dempster, H. (1993) 'Child sexual abuse: the child's perspective', in Ferguson, H., Gilligan, R. and Torode, R. (eds) *Surviving Childhood Adversity: Issues for Policy and Practice*, Dublin: Social Studies Press, Trinity College Dublin.

Thompson, F. (1945) *Lark Rise to Candleford*, London: Penguin.

The Times (1996) 'Disruptive pupil cured by learning with mother', 25 May, p. 4.

Tizard, B., Blatchford, P., Burke, J., Farquhar, C. and Plewis, I. (1988) *Young Children at School in the Inner City*, London: Thomas Coram Research Unit/Lawrence Erlbaum.

Tomlinson, S. (1981) *Educational Subnormality: A Study in Decision-Making*, London: Routledge & Kegan Paul.

Tomlinson, S. (1982) *A Sociology of Special Education*, London: Routledge & Kegan Paul,

Townsend, P. (1991) *The Poor and Poorer: A Statistical Report on Changes in the Living Standards of Rich and Poor in the United Kingdom 1979–1989*, Bristol: Department of Social Policy and Social Planning, University of Bristol.

Union of the Physically Impaired Against Segregation (1976) *Fundamental Principles of Disability*, London: UPIAS.

Veljanovski, C. (1990) Foreword to de Jasay, A. *Market Socialism: A Scrutiny of 'This Square Circle'*, London: Institute for Economic Affairs.

Waddell, A. (1996) 'Oldham Young Carers Project: Meeting the Needs of Young Carers in Oldham?' Unpublished MA thesis, Huddersfield: University of Huddersfield.

Walker, A. (1996) *Young Carers and their Families: A Survey carried out by the Social Survey Division of the Office for National Statistics on behalf of the Department of Health*, London: The Stationery Office.

Walker, T. (1994) 'Educating children in the public care: a strategic approach', *Oxford Review of Education*, 20, 3, pp. 329–47.

Wallace, W. (1995) 'He ain't heavy, he's my father', *Times Educational Supplement*, 3 March, pp. 3–4.

Wallerstein, J. and Kelly, J. (1980) *Surviving the Breakup – How Parents and Children Cope with Divorce*, London: Grant McIntyre.

Walmsley, R., Howard, L. and White, S. (1992) *The National Prison Survey 1991: Main Findings*, Home Office Research Study 128, London: HMSO.

Walrond-Skinner, S. (1976) *Family Therapy: The Treatment of Natural Systems*, London: Routledge & Kegan Paul.

Warnock, M. (1992) *Special Case in Need of Reform*, Observer Schools Report, 18 October, p. 3.

Webb, R. (1994) *After the Deluge: Changing Roles and Responsibilities in the Primary School. Final Report of Research commissioned by the Association of Teachers and Lecturers*, London: Association of Teachers and Lecturers.

Weddell, K. (1993) *Special Needs Education: The Next 25 Years*, London: National Commission on Education.

Weir, A. (1994) 'Split decisions', *Community Care*, 1–7 December, p. 18.

Weir, S. and Hall, W. (1994) *Ego Trip: Extra-governmental Organisations in the UK and their Accountability: The Democratic Audit of the UK*, London: Charter 88 Trust.

Wells, G. (1984) *Language Development in the Pre-School Years*, Cambridge: Cambridge University Press.

Werner, E. (1990) 'Protective factors and individual resilience', in Meisels, S. and Shonkoff, J. (eds) *Handbook of Early Childhood Intervention*. Cambridge: Cambridge University Press.

West Yorkshire Police and West Yorkshire Local Education Authorities (1988) *Responsible Citizenship Schools/Police: Curriculum Liaison*, Wakefield: West Yorkshire Police and West Yorkshire Local Education Authorities.

Westcott, H. (1993) *Abuse of Children and Adults with Disabilities*, London: NSPCC.

Westcott, H. and Clément, M. (1992) *NSPCC Experience of Child Abuse in Residential Care and Educational Placements: Results of a Survey*, London: NSPCC.

Westcott, H. and Cross, M. (1996) *This Far and No Further: Towards Ending the Abuse of Disabled Children*, Birmingham: Venture Press.

Westwood, S. (1990) 'Racism, black masculinity and the politics of space', in Hearn, J. and Morgan, D. H. J. (eds) *Men, Masculinities and Social Theory*, London and Winchester: Unwin Hyman.

White, C. (1996) 'New Order', *Community Care*, 2–8 May, pp. 16–17.

Whitehead, M. (1996) 'Plea for tougher law on truancy', *Times Educational Supplement* 31 May, p. 2.

Whitney, B. (1994) *The Truth About Truancy*, London: Kogan Page.

Whitney, I. and Smith, P. K. (1993) 'A survey of the nature and extent of bullying in junior, middle and secondary schools', *Educational Research*, 35, 1, pp. 2–25.

Whitty, G. and Menter, I. (1989) 'Lessons of Thatcherism: education policy in England and Wales 1979–1988', *Journal of Law and Society*, 16, 1, pp. 42–64.

Whitty, G. and Menter, I. (1991). 'The progress of restructuring', in Coulby, D. and Bash, L. (eds) *The 1988 Education Reform Act: Conflict and Contradiction*, London: Cassell.

Whyte, J. (1983) *Beyond the Wendy House: Sex Role Stereotyping in Primary Schools*, York: Longman School Council Resources Unit.

Williams *v* Eady (1893) 10, TLR 41, CA.

Willis, P. (1977) *Learning to Labour: How Working Class Kids Get Working Class Jobs*, Aldershot: Saxton House.

Winter, M. (1983) 'Remedial education', in Whyld, J. (ed.) *Sexism in the Secondary Curriculum*, London: Harper & Row.

Wood, L. (1992) *Leeds Children of Parents with Schizophrenia*, Leeds: Research and Development Group, Leeds City Council, Department of Social Services.

Woods, P., Bagley, C. and Glatter, R. (1996) 'Dynamics of competition – the effects of local competitive arenas in schools', in Pole, C. and Chawla-Duggan, R. (eds) *Reshaping Education in the 1990s: Perspectives on Secondary Schooling*, London: Falmer Press.

Wright, J. (1990) 'Out of school', *New Society*, 9 February, pp. 26–7.

Yorkshire Post (1994) 'Teachers take tough line over classroom violence', 8 April, p. 6.

INDEX

absenteeism, school
  authorised, 79, 80
  categorisation, 79–80, 84
  and children in care, 48
  and performance tables, 28
  reasons for, 5
  and 'whole school approach',
    84, 85
  and young carers, 66
  see also truancy
abuse, child, 112–27
  case conferences, 122–3, 124
  by children, 114
  definition, 114
  and disabled children, 99,
    115–17, 126
  and domestic violence, 118–19
  identification of children,
    115–18
  informing parents of, 121–2
  mandate to prevent, 112–13
  need for avoidance of
    subordination of women
    in preventing, 119–20, 125
  opportunities for locating at
    school, 113
  parenting courses for fathers,
    125
  recording and reporting of, 120–1
  responding to by teachers,
    120–4
  safety training, 125
  in schools, 113–15
  schools' role in preventing of,
    124–7
  sexual, 14, 114, 116, 124
  and social services, 38, 43
  teachers role in locating, 10

and young carers, 70
ADD (Attention Deficit
  Disorder), 105
African Caribbeans, 20, 21–2,
  22–3, 104
Ahmad, B., 36
Aitken, Robert, 6, 7
Alderson, K., 107
Aldridge, J. and Becker, S., 65
'Amanda', 115
Asians, 21, 22
Assisted Places Scheme, 24–5
Association of Teachers and
  Lecturers, 38
attendance, school, 74–100
  categorisation of absenteeism,
    79–80, 84
  and children in care, 48
  and education welfare officers,
    41, 86
  enforcement of, 5–7, 80
  and GEST initiatives, 83–4,
    85–6
  introduction of computerised
    registration system, 84–5
  law and policy on, 79–80
  and Leeds adjournment
    scheme, 8, 37, 46, 70, 82
  and performance tables, 74, 80
  prevalence and patterns, 74–5
  reasons for absenteeism, 5
  and School Attendance
    Officers, 6
  and state intervention in family
    life, 7–9
  and 'whole school approach',
    84, 85
  see also truancy